If you're stressed out and looking for answers to your challenges, this book will give you the right questions. If from time to time you "lose it," this book will help you "find it." The most useful book of the decade! **–John Miller, CEO, Denny's Restaurants**

Peppered with personal anecdotes, illuminating stories, vulnerable authenticity and raw emotion. It's a life-affirming, uplifting and entertaining read. I recommend it highly. **–Doug Kirkpatrick, author: *Beyond Empowerment – The Age of the Self-Managed Organization***

Any coach, mentor or individual interested in bringing their best to high performance situations should get this book. **–Joshua Rosenthal MA ED, Supervisor, Cultural Development, Colorado Rockies Baseball Team**

Valid clinical insights from nothing more than acute observation of human dynamics and cultural patterns. This book underlines, simplifies and highlights what it is that people really need—experiential confidence in relationship to the challenges of being human. **–John Souza, LMFT, DMFT, BF**

Demonstrates why presence is a fundamental competency of leadership—guiding any leader to stress smarter, to evolve in tandem as stresses arise and to handle the complexities of work and life with useful action. **–Fred Scarborough, CFRE, President, Arkansas Children's Foundation**

A truly authentic and entertaining narrative. This is a must read that surprises you with its simplicity. – **Desiree Bombenon, President and CEO, Sure Call Contact Centers**

An insightful and inspiring read that provides a revelatory analysis of the lingering effects of trauma and exposes the truth behind stress. **–Kristy Hart, Senior Account Associate, CB Insurance**

It's been more beneficial to me than many years of therapy. Maybe that's because there is a dash of humor and no invoice. **–Keith F. Mobley, P.E., G.E., President, Northern Geotechnical Engineering**

The tools in this book serve as a guide for tapping into our social brains and developing new neural pathways that serve us well. **–Linda Roszak Burton, Certified Neuroleadership Institute Coach, International Coaching Federation ACC Accreditation**

Packed with both the motivation and the means to launch into the life and the career you were meant for, but didn't believe was possible. **–Joe Ward, Director of Customer Support and Services, Sage**

What he teaches has not only expanded my income, it's also improved my marriage. I highly recommend you give his book your attention. **–Justin Bentley, National Sales Director, Telcom National**

Rick is both entertaining and challenging in a way that makes the reader rethink what we all have learned as we grew from innocent and optimistic child into doubting adult. **–Terry Dwyer, EVP, Managing Director of Tax and Transportation, First Advantage Corp**

Wonderfully engaging writing as he weaves his personal stories with scientific research and expert advice. **–Dr. Geoffrey Carr, R. Psych, author:** *Making Happiness – for You, Your Relationships, and Your Children*

Rick shows us how to uplift ourselves and help others to live with confidence. It's a must read. **–Ashif Mawji, Hon. Colonel, Canadian Armed Forces**

This book was a needed wake-up call to exit the well-traveled superhighway of my old ways of thinking. **–Rich Pflederer, CEO, Medical Management Innovations**

A beautifully crafted machine that converts complex research into simple tools that we can use right now, in a modern, chaotic world. **–Thomas W. Blackburn, PE, GE, President, Blackburn Consulting**

With humor and insight Rick helps us keep our potential in view and our confidence afloat as we navigate the potholes of everyday life. **–Michael White, Business Development Manager, Activate Healthcare**

Provides essential tools for illuminating the blind spots that we suffer from and for increasing confidence through the subtle nuances of our behavior. **–Sam Sanregret, President, Capital Lumber**

A clear analysis and simple tools, along with an open-hearted perspective, offer a powerful antidote to despair, and a reminder to readers that change lies within grasp. **–Rob Schmidt, Co-Director, Tayu Meditation Center**

An instruction manual for building your own adventure experience without leaving home. **–Tom Benson, Chief Experience Officer, WildPlay Element Parks**

A useful reminder that I can take much greater charge of my experience of stress rather than being a victim of it. **–BJ Lingren, President, eLogger Inc.**

One of the most compelling arguments for professional play that I've ever run across. Prepare to get the best from your inner child. **–Zachary Q. Dungca, LMFTA, Play Therapist**

This book is founded in solid-neuroscience, yet written in a simple story-telling style. **–Deborah Zelinsky, O.D., Founder, Mind-Eye Connection**

Translates the neuroscience, psychology and the spirit of our human nature into an immediately actionable guide for increasing confidence in our personal and work lives. **–Paul Eisen, Head of User Experience, PwC Canada**

OTHER BOOKS BY RICK LEWIS

The Perfection of Nothing: Reflections on Spiritual Practice (Hohm Press, 2000)

You Have the Right to Remain Silent: Bringing Meditation to Life (Hohm Press, 2002)

7 Rules You Were Born to Break: How Intelligent Misbehavior Can Help You and Your Organization Thrive (Break a Rule Publishing, 2010)

Sounding the Alarm on Business as Usual: Transforming Work with Intelligent Misbehavior (Break a Rule Publishing, 2012) Available at www.breakarule.com

CONFIDENT UNDER PRESSURE

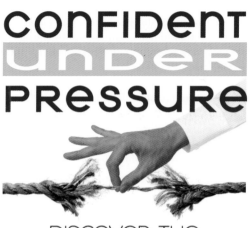

DISCOVER THE HIDDEN ADVANTAGES OF STRESS

RICK LEWIS

HOHM PRESS
CHINO VALLEY, ARIZONA

Cover Design and Interior Graphics: Rick Lewis
Interior Design and Layout: Becky Fulker, Kubera Book Design, Prescott, Arizona

Library of Congress Cataloging-in-Publication Data

Names: Lewis, Rick, 1961- author.
Title: Confident under pressure : discover the hidden advantages of stress / Rick Lewis.
Description: Chino Valley, Arizona : Hohm Press, 2018. | Includes index.
Identifiers: LCCN 2018002543 | ISBN 9781942493402 (trade pbk. : alk. paper)
Subjects: LCSH: Stress management--Popular works. | Stress (Physiology)--Popular works.
Classification: LCC RA785 .L49 2018 | DDC 616.9/8--dc23
LC record available at https://lccn.loc.gov/2018002543

Hohm Press
P.O. Box 4410
Chino Valley, AZ 86323
800-381-2700
http://www.hohmpress.com

This book was printed in China.

Previous ISBN: 978-0-9866730-5-4

FOR Lee
SOURCE OF CONFIDENCE

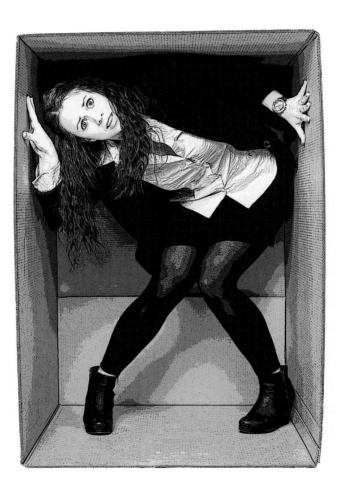

contents

FOREWORD

As a union President for the Fraternal Order of Police, to say I understand and experience stress would be the understatement of a lifetime. Thank God for Rick Lewis and his book *Confident Under Pressure*. The lifeline was thrown and I received it. Much like being in attendance at a Rick Lewis presentation, I found myself transformed to a place and a time where I was able to take a break from the rigors of everyday life and the pressures of politics, contract negotiations, disciplinary hearings and the occasional nail biting life or death scenario that is, of course, a part of the life of the first responders I represent.

In my spare time, I lead a critical incident team and specialize in peer support and stress. The key goals that involve our personal health are essential and must be achieved especially in the law enforcement / first responder fields, where finishing our careers in one piece physically is our goal. Next, we must be able to handle the stress of the job emotionally. We must deal with each critical situation and survive the moment. However, we must do as Rick advises, remembering that we are "first *responders*" and not simply "reactors." Otherwise, the effects of years of cumulative stress as we cope with these intense situations can and do take a heavy toll on many of us. The impact of stress is well documented. We have, thankfully moved far beyond the days of stuffing our emotions deep in the filing cabinet of life.

As Rick teaches us so effectively throughout this book, we have the choice to handle stress on our own terms if we're proactive about it, or we can be left dealing with stress on its terms if we try to ignore it. The latter is obviously far more destructive. As Rick accurately promises, *Confident Under Pressure* details how to use and to even *design* stress that works to one's advantage. We can learn useful ways to engage with our stressors so that we may thrive and enjoy our lives. If we utilize the lessons within this wonderful book, there will be laughter involved as we not only survive, but succeed in distressing and re-engaging.

Take Rick's lead and allow him to teach you just how you should and could be properly tackling the stressors of your life. With humor and a self-guided tour of your own limiting past and possible future, Rick will give you surefire guidance to live, laugh and de-stress in an honest and true way. And trust me, he'll provide you with an amazing read that will entertain the whole way through!

Michael J. Saxe
President, Lodge 145 M.C.S.O.
Florida State Lodge
Fraternal Order of Police

PART ONE

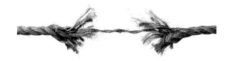

5 REACTIONS THAT ARE KILLING YOUR CONFIDENCE

A STRESSED OUT CITIZEN JUST LIKE YOU

Would you like to know how to live more confidently and effectively, even under pressure?

Of course you would.

Well, you've come to the right place, because I'm a stressed-out citizen just like you who has made his living in the last twenty years by walking smack into the middle of stressful situations and making the best of them. I've done a lot of thinking, research, and hands-on experimenting with how to maintain confidence in situations where we are most likely to lose it. That's really what this book is about: *how you can remain confident under pressure and even turn stress to your advantage instead of becoming its victim.*

My experience with being up against a great deal of stress in my life has led to the discovery of some unique and innovative ways for handling it. As an author, speaker, and entertainer, I've appeared before one million people, demonstrating and talking about how to handle stress more confidently. I do this by first creating and then resolving stressful situations. I know, sounds crazy, huh? More on that in a minute.

Before I share my secrets, however, we need to face the current reality of our stressful lives and the ways we react to being under pressure now. At the risk of having you put this book down after you read the next sentence, I'll start the ball rolling by telling you this: Today I threw a potato at the wall because it was taking too long to cook.

I was home alone with my six-year-old, who was having a hunger meltdown. We were behind on our grocery shopping, and he burned through the remaining carrot sticks while I tried to get the frickin' potato ready, but the thing just wouldn't cook! My wife was out, so as the head of my household in that moment I did the only logical thing. I took charge by pulling that potato out of the oven and throwing it against the wall.

Now we all run into frustrations in the course of our daily routines. That's one thing. When those frustrations build up, however, and we're not properly digesting them, we can wind up taking actions that are not particularly useful or appropriate in dealing with the present moment.

I'll be the first to admit, this wasn't all about the potato. Given the absurdity of my actions, you might conclude that I'm stressed, and you'd be right. As a professional meeting presenter with three kids, traveling frequently for business in two countries while navigating multiple tax laws, bouncing between time zones when I need to be at my best on demand in front of thousands of people, handling all the administrative hassles that involve servicing clients as a traveling consultant, billing in multiple currencies, authoring and publishing books as I go, and acknowledging the fact that I put myself out of a job each time I successfully deliver for my clients—yes, I'm stressed.

So, pressure is a big part of my life, and it's not going to go away. Now, you may find this hard to believe after the spud confession, but the ability to perform confidently under pressure is actually how I earn my living.

Getting Booed on the Stage of Life

Many years ago I was contacted by the Fort St. John Oilman's Association in the far north of British Columbia, Canada, about an event they were planning. They required entertainment for five hundred association members—oil field and rig workers—for their winter celebration. A contract was signed, and before I knew it I was bouncing way up north on a little prop plane to the small, snowy town where the sun shines for about six hours a day in the winter months.

My performance would take place at the local high school on a stage that was at one end of the cafeteria following the group's celebration dinner. I stood ready behind the red velvet curtain as the announcement was made that it was time for the evening's entertainment. The men were full of energy, excited, and vocally enthusiastic—until the emcee asked them to put their hands together for juggler Rick Lewis.

No one had bothered to mention to me that the only form of entertainment provided to these men in the previous twenty years had involved a boom box and a person of the opposite sex trained in the slow and methodic removal of various pieces of clothing.

The curtain went up as the loud booing of the crowd filled the entire auditorium. I stood there as they jeered, wondering what would happen next. From halfway to the back of the hall, one of the men threw his spoon, which landed with a ping on the wooden stage where I was standing. There was a pause, and a moment later several hundred more spoons were launched into the air, like shrapnel from an exploding bomb. The spoons clattered to stillness on the stage, and then all the men went silent, waiting to see what I would do.

Life is full of such moments, though mostly not quite so dramatic, where we are faced with the choice between crumbling under pressure or rising to the occasion of our challenges. I remember my heart pounding and my mind racing, looking for an option as to how to proceed. I knew that if I panicked in the face of their taunt, I would have no chance of being able to proceed with the show. I had no more than a few seconds to communicate who I was and what I had to offer, or lose that audience for good.

I stared out at the audience as the tension peaked and the crowd waited to see how I would react to their protest. Channeling all the adrenaline that was coursing through my body, I sprang into the air, performed a full backflip, feet to feet, and again stood still, looking out at the crowd. (It wasn't my first backflip.)

There was another moment of silence before the entire group erupted into applause and cheers. I had earned their respect and was able to successfully complete the performance.

Likely, you can remember a time yourself when the creative tension of an uncertain situation drew forth the best you had to offer. In my case, every one of those oilfield workers left there smiling, laughing, and slapping each other on the back in a spirit of camaraderie. As you know, it's a great feeling when dicey situations work out, but I had to stretch well beyond my usual comfort zone to facilitate that result.

I've gotten pretty good over the years at navigating such challenges and have learned some things about how to capitalize on the presence of stress and turn it to everyone's advantage—as long as there aren't any root vegetables in the audience. Now I regularly consult with the top executives of Fortune 500 companies to help them—not only to deal with the stress of delivering successful events for their organizations, but to educate and inspire attendees to find confident footing when under pressure at work.

Briefly, here's how I do it.

A REALLY BAD WAITER

What's more annoying than terrible service? In our cushy modern-day lives, it's often the worst part of our day. It used to be that getting eaten by a tiger could be the worst part of our day. Now, it's when we're not getting served or attended to the way we expect. The funny part is, we react to our small daily challenges in much the same way as we do to the prospect of being mauled by a wild animal: by getting really stressed and losing our capacity for effective and confident action.

As a speaker and meeting presenter, I draw attention to this phenomenon. I dress up identically to the serving staff at a corporate event, and I pretend to be an inept waiter who gets more and more clumsy, odd, and eccentric. By the end of the meal, everybody is exchanging perplexed looks and whispering about how this server ever got his job and how he's keeping it. I can see them wondering what they should do next: get the manager, or confront me directly?

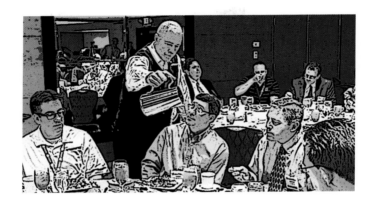

And it's not just the attendees who are challenged by the situation. It's a theatrically stressful circumstance that the guests and I navigate together. The experience of having a few hundred people level their silent judgments at me and being at the effect of their stares, looks, and snide comments about my abilities is always stressful for me, too. No matter how many times I've done it successfully, my confidence always gets a little shaken by these interactions.

Not only that, but the resident servers and banquet managers have to play along, too—answering questions in a credible manner for guests who want to know what's going on without giving away that I'm an act. I brief them in advance on how to handle that challenge and how to function as a team of co-conspirators, all while they deliver their usual superior service. So they have to muster confidence in playing along with an unusual and unfamiliar routine.

Sounds stressful, right? Well, it is, but before the event I express my utmost faith in the staff's ability to play along. I tell them I'm happy to step in if they feel overly challenged by the reactions of a guest, I give clear directions, and I thank them for helping me out.

Despite the stress involved, the staff always loves it! The event becomes one of the banquet team's most memorable experiences at the hotel, and they talk about it for years to come. In fact, it's *because* of the stress involved that the incident becomes such a satisfying experience. I'll expand on this point in a bit.

Eventually, I'm introduced by the facility manager, who I also enroll to cooperate with the routine. He or she comes to the microphone and says, "Folks, we're really sorry, we pride ourselves on our service here, but today we had a new server who was very nervous and apparently has made some of you uncomfortable. I've asked him to come out and apologize, so please give him a minute of your time."

Because most of my presentations take place in the impeccable environments of the world's top hotels and conference centers, this baffles the usual attendee even further. The stress of my poor service and what to do about it is turned up another notch as they watch the terrified waiter edge his way out of the service door. I stumble up on stage to "apologize," looking like the least confident person in the world. And it's not all an act. I really *am* nervous, and I use the pressure that I'm actually feeling to portray a convincingly petrified character.

I draw the audience a bit further into the ruse as I stammer for words, then suddenly reveal to the crowd that they've been set up, that I'm their speaker, and that this has all been for the purpose of entering into a learning conversation. As a dawning wave of recognition ripples across the room, there are groans of laughter, and there's also the palpable sense of relief that it was all a gag. What it sets us up for is a dialogue about what happens to our confidence when we're faced with challenging circumstances—personally or professionally.

Based on the experience they've just had, I invite the audience members to examine what their default habits are in stressful situations and what reactions arise when things aren't going as planned. Some tried to ignore the evidence and deny there was a problem, others got insulted and demanded better treatment, some just shot dirty looks in my direction or complained to a neighbor without saying a word to me—the person they had the issue with.

With the reference point of what has just occurred, these event participants are able to gain some insights about their tendencies in the face of pressure and how they typically react when they're on the receiving end of unexpected circumstances or behavior.

THREE CONFLICT STYLES

My surprise waiter theater is a useful frame through which we can study the dynamics of conflict. In daily life we are always being confronted by a conflict between what we want and what we actually get in real life.

Diane Musho Hamilton is both a Zen teacher and a professional mediator. In her recent book *Everything Is Workable*, she explains how most individuals fixate upon one of three conflict styles. When conflict is present, most of us default to one of three strategies:

1. Avoid

2. Accommodate

3. Compete

Imagine having a bad waiter slop water around your table just as you take your seat for dinner. How do you respond to the intrusion? Probably in one of these three ways:

1. Pretending there isn't any problem and trying to ignore the alarming behavior

2. Bending over backward to adapt to the offender's shortcomings while trying at the same time to calm down others around you who have been offended

3. Taking the poor service as a personal attack and becoming verbally or visually aggressive

After participating in this piece of theater, most individuals are easily able to identify their conflict style and see how ineffective it is to rely on a single, set approach to managing our challenges. We can see that such reactions arise from feeling unprepared to cope with our stress.

Right there in the middle of the meeting we replay the circumstance by assigning one guest at each table to act as the bad waiter. He or she picks up a water pitcher and replicates the terrible, sloppy service I just delivered.

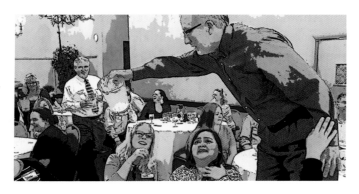

The tension and stress that was previously experienced is suddenly transformed into creative delight. Above, one gentleman mounts a chair to challenge my status as the highest-pouring waiter in the world.

Another decides that drinking directly from the pitcher before providing refills to his table will lighten things up.

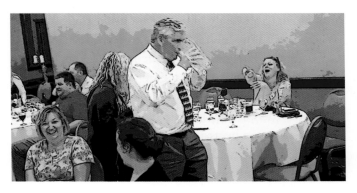

All we've done so far is introduce two keys to living with more enjoyment and confidence: awareness and the permission to play.

When we take back our inalienable right to live with both presence of the current moment and our opportunity to play within it, we have a different experience. What started out as a stressful circumstance has now become a ton of fun for everyone. Playfulness is an essential ingredient if we truly want to consider how we can act with greater effectiveness when the unexpected lands on our plate in daily life.

In addition to awareness and playfulness, we need to take a fresh look at what stress really is and where it actually comes from.

HOW MUCH STRESS can YOU HanDLe?

Data from a National Health Interview Survey based on responses from millions of adults concluded that those who reported they had a lot of stress *and also believed that stress impacted their health* had a 43 percent increased risk of premature death! [1]

Whoa.

Translation: How we *expect* stress to affect us is a huge determinant in how stress *will* affect us. And, culturally, there are predictable patterns to our stress expectations. The Holmes and Rahe Stress Scale is an analysis of circumstances and life events that most people experience as being stressful. Things like divorce, death, accidents, job changes, moving to a different city, and surgery are on that list. Yet many of the heroic stories that inspire us about leaders, athletes, or even everyday parents who overcome chronic stressors all depict individuals who found a way to respond to massive challenges in an extraordinary way, rather than in a usual manner. All of these stress champions have one thing in common: an unusual mastery over their perception and attention.

So, rather than stress being some objective measure of difficulty, stress is more a measure of the disparity between what we *think* we can handle and what we're actually given to work with. This is a major key to predicting where we will lose our confidence or maintain it.

I believe that what we think we can handle is often heavily influenced by personal precedent. For example, if a schoolmate teases us in front of the whole class in second grade after we innocently declare our affection to him or her, we might not consciously remember the episode. Yet, we'll be baffled later in life as to why we're terrified of intimacy or plagued by trust issues.

Our minds make judgments about our own lives in a fashion similar to a court of law. If there is a preexisting judgment that applies to the current circumstance we're facing, that precedent will sway the opinion of the court. Our mind, in this case, is the court. The precedent is our trauma. (The schoolmate teasing.) The final judgment is, "You can't handle this!" (vulnerability or intimacy in relationship). In short, the trauma that sets these precedents in our formative childhood years is often responsible for the loss of confidence we experience as adults.

We now reference the way we failed to handle past stress as children to assess the likelihood of whether we can handle it now!

Obviously, this is not a fair or accurate measurement of our adult capacity, but because our files have not been updated, we buy the outdated assessment, and our confidence is unnecessarily undermined. This explains how in some situations a perfectly capable grownup can be reduced to paralysis in the face of simple tasks such as speaking to a small group of people, asking for a date, requesting a raise, or needing to take a spider out of the house. The past colors our perception of what we can handle in the present. When that process goes on in us unconsciously, we wind up *reacting* to the stresses of our lives rather than usefully *responding* to them.

WE'RE ALL BORN CONFIDENT

What's the difference between reacting and responding? To answer that question, we need to talk about childhood and the behavior of kids in general. Here are some actual test questions that were recently posed to young students at school and the real answers they provided in response.[2]

The first question: *What ended in 1896?*
One child answered: 1895.

The second question: *The first cells were probably…?*
Another child answered: *Lonely.*
The third question: *The strongest force on earth is…?*
Another child answered: *Love.*

Like me, I'm guessing you were probably uplifted in some way by these answers. I have a theory about why we enjoy these responses. They demonstrate confidence under pressure!

All children everywhere are born with a freedom of spirit and a creative capacity that can shine forth when the pressure is on. What parent among us hasn't been baffled by the ingenuity and fearlessness of our children in the face of limits, boundaries, and challenges? If we're lucky, we preserve some measure of that spunk as we enter our adult lives. Many of us, however, have distanced ourselves from the kind of confidence required to be at our best, so simply demonstrated by the responses of these schoolchildren. Instead, we're dealing with the baggage of minor, and sometimes major, traumas. Not knowing what else to do with it, we're dragging the load behind us into every meeting, relationship, and family outing, undermining our confidence in the process.

There is a lot of talk about confidence these days in the circles of personal growth and even professional and organizational development. We're just using fancier concepts to describe it. There is talk of *mindfulness, agility, innovation, resilience, creativity, productivity, leadership, disruption, conflict resolution*—all of which map directly to confidence. And a good case can be made that the bedrock components of organizational excellence—teamwork, communication, integrity, culture, and vision—all suffer when confidence is missing.

The test answers the kids gave are entertaining as well as instructive. The delight we find in their responses comes from the creativity, authenticity, and courage they demonstrate in response to a stressful circumstance. We have all experienced the stress of being tested. Yet, the freedom expressed by the children's answers defies the stress patterns of most adults, where we tend to repress the range of our responsiveness when we're challenged, rather than increase it.

Similarly, a great deal of what inspires us about historical or modern-day heroes involves their ability to freely, innovatively, and confidently respond when the stakes are high. That's what these schoolchildren are demonstrating: the potential to offer a confident response even in the stressful moments of life.

Here's an image of one of those proud and creative answers marked "wrong." It epitomizes the current state of our human affairs. It explains how the natural confidence that we're connected to as children is discouraged over time and leaves us living less than

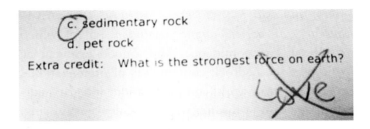

c. Sedimentary rock

d. pet rock

Extra credit: What is the strongest force on earth?

Love

joyfully in our adult lives. It explains why we don't thrive in our work, because we're taught, for example, that love is not how we succeed. In fact, it's how we earn a big red X for our authentic responsiveness and passion.

While our confidence cannot technically be taken away by someone else, children especially can be compelled to distance themselves from it when their free responses are met with disapproval by the adults they depend upon for guidance and for love. The next time this child is asked, "What is the strongest force on earth?," she is going to consciously or unconsciously recall the painful experience of being corrected about her view of love. She will doubt her natural intelligence and give an answer that satisfies her need for relational safety. For a child, betraying her feelings to preserve her physical and emotional safety is an instinctually appropriate response in the moment. Sadly, however, this child is likely to fall into a self-doubting *pattern* when in the future she is asked any question by a teacher—and later by employers, friends, and colleagues. What she has now internalized, backed by the force of negative emotion, is a *stress precedent*. A stress precedent is a strong belief about what we can or can't handle. She'll now be on the lookout for patterns, tones, moods, colors, smells, and cues that might help her to anticipate and protect herself from future rejection. This will become an attention pattern that feels normal and unremarkable to her, despite the degree of tension and self-limitation it introduces into her life.

Trauma Is Reactive, Confidence Is Responsive

So we're born with confidence, yet most of us have been conditioned into reactive behavior: taking actions and making decisions that arise out of being in the grip of a past pain. *The unconscious recall of past pain prompts evasive measures to avoid the repeated experience of a previous wounding.* That's the definition of a reaction.

Have you ever reacted in an automatic and unthinking way when you wished you could have responded thoughtfully or usefully instead? Have you ever silenced your authenticity? Have you ever backed away from a challenge—or even a wonderful opportunity—because the idea of engaging it was just too stressful?

Your answers put you in good company with the rest of the human race. We all struggle to respond confidently to the challenges and opportunities of our lives.

- We all wish we could make clear, timely decisions, rather than doubting the right course of action.

- We wish we could trust ourselves to speak up and communicate our perspective instead of muzzling ourselves out of fear.

- We all wish to take action on the wonderful opportunities that show up in our lives instead of hesitating and missing out.

So why do we fail so often to achieve these wishes? Perhaps because responsiveness requires practice and a significant intentional effort. The first step of this concerted effort requires simply being able to see our reactivity as it and how it routinely plays out in our day-to-day habits.

Red Hawk is the author of *Self Observation: The Awakening of Conscience, an Owner's Manual.* In the book, he describes the essential role that self observation plays in educating ourselves about our existing tendencies, rather than blindly rushing forward in an attempt to change them.

> *...the inner observer can begin to predict the habitual behavior of the mammal instrument, the body, and be prepared for it. It learns the patterns.*

It knows itself. This is my only hope for becoming more conscious and not at the mercy of habit; if I see the habit often enough, say 10,000 times or more, then I can begin to predict where, when, and how it will manifest exactly as it has so many times before, and I may be prepared before it arises. I may be able to choose another course. Certainly I may be able to view the habits more objectively. In this way, I can cease to be always a victim of my own habits. (p. 3)

By default, our collective history of small or significant traumas rules our behavior because they are dominant in our memory.[3] Those traumatic associations trigger automatic and familiar reactions that are comforting and feel good in the moment. Our reactions are like triple-chocolate cake, unguarded and unclaimed on the counter of an empty kitchen. It's only later that we regret indulging them.

Responding, on the other hand, requires that we retrain ourselves

- to clearly see our automatic behaviors.

- to identify alternatives to those old behaviors.

- to exercise those alternatives in the heat of a stressful moment.

So here's your own test question: For any adult who wants to reclaim a full measure of confidence related to the challenges of life—what is the strongest force on earth?

The answer is *practice.*

As a confidence coach, my intention is to share with you exactly what you need to practice in order to live with confidence under pressure. I'm excited to share the things you can do to handle stress more effectively. Given the fact that you're still reading, you're probably anxious to know what those things are. First, however, we need to understand that the difference between making use of stress that shows up unavoidably and actually *creating* stress for ourselves unnecessarily! This falls squarely into the self observation category described by Red Hawk. Our first task is to take a look at the ways we *unconsciously and unnecessarily increase the stress we're suffering from.* We need to begin by *stopping,* or *refraining from,* old reactive patterns before we try to add anything new to our behavioral repertoire.

Past traumas lead to present stress, which leads to shaky confidence. If we can stop reacting to the past, we can free ourselves to live confidently in the present. Interrupting the stress patterns that we habitually reinforce can break the link between those old traumas and the confidence we need in the present.

How We Make Our Stress Worse

Several years ago I wound up in my doctor's office to ask him if I might be having a heart attack because my chest was hurting so badly. I was expecting that I might be ushered into an urgent care unit for a battery of special tests. Instead, my doctor handed me a reading list of books on stress. I learned that I was far from alone in suffering from its effects.

According to a resource provided by the National Center for Biotechnology Information, emotional stress contributes to the six leading causes of death: heart disease, cancer, lung ailments, accidental injuries, cirrhosis of the liver, and suicide. And an estimated 75 percent of physician office visits are for stress-related problems and complaints.[4] Much of our stress is occupationally related. The workplace doesn't just produce goods and services, it's the manufacturing center for stress in the world. One researcher has put the rough estimate of spending on stress-related healthcare at 300 billion dollars annually.[5]

And all of the above represents only the medically correlated effects of stress.

Another price we pay for stress is failed or even nonexistent communication. The National Institute of Mental Health reports that 74 percent of people suffer from speech anxiety.[6] We can safely assume that a lot of things aren't getting said! What that means is that stress is not just leading to death, it's killing our ability to fully enjoy and participate in life and work.

We might conclude at this point that all we need to do is eliminate the things that are causing stress. What I've learned, however, is that the elimination of what seems to be causing us stress is not the only (or even the best) way to address our problem. Recall the National Health Interview Survey I mentioned earlier in which those who reported they had a lot of stress, and also believed that stress impacted their health, had a 43 percent increased risk of premature death over those who didn't believe that stress had an effect on their health. This data clearly demonstrates that the presence of external challenges isn't really the issue. What determines our experience is how we *expect* those challenges will impact us, what kind of stress precedents we've formed previously in our lives, and whether we react poorly or respond usefully to the real situations we face.

Reducing external triggers may in fact be a reasonable course of action as part of a stress management program. However, much of our stress comes from past trauma, and *working to modify present conditions doesn't eliminate the intrusive nature of our past experiences*. In many cases, we have to leave present conditions as they are, stop trying to manipulate them, and instead work on changing *ourselves* and the habitual nature of our reactions. If we want to stop making our stress worse, we have to ask ourselves a question different from how can I make my stress go away? In fact, this whole book is an answer to the following question:

How could someone use the presence of real life challenges to access the root of their trauma, eliminate the disabling expectations of stress, and turn the pressures of ordinary life into fuel for growth?

Yes, I am suggesting that the presence of stress, properly processed and digested, could actually be a means of *growing* one's confidence. The key is to make a distinction between the actual challenges of our lives and the ways in which we compound our stress disproportionately to the issues at hand. We need to see where we get triggered into unconscious patterns of stress reactivity that, ironically, make our stress worse.

Cultivating a New Perspective

I've seen these unconscious patterns of self-induced stress in others firsthand through the accidental sociology study I have inadvertently conducted over the years I've spent imitating an inept waiter. I've carefully observed tens of thousands of people as they've had to deal with the nonlife-threatening reality of a bad waiter, and I've seen the contrasting behaviors of happy and unhappy people again and again.

Happy people become present and curious when things aren't going as planned or aren't living up to their expectations. They take responsibility for their dissatisfaction and pursue practical avenues for change while considering the experience of others. Unhappy people jump to conclusions about what is actually happening, make assumptions, and assign blame—prior to admitting that their negative experience might have a good deal to do with their own perceptions, beyond the situation at hand. If I'm pouring water sloppily at a table where eight people are seated, four might be looking at me with curiosity and amusement, while the other four are insulted and alarmed by exactly the same actions.

The peak performers, successful leaders, top producers, and personally happy people of the world are those who take unusual and unfamiliar circumstances as their cue to

- become more present,

- get more interested,

- and delay their judgments about what's wrong with a given situation.

When I think back to the episode with the oilfield workers in Northern Canada, I sometimes wonder what would have happened if I had panicked in the face of their taunts. It was a close call. Things could have gone in either direction, which is true with a lot of the best comedy. It's also true with the best of life, that to achieve those best moments we have to expose ourselves to elements that are outside of our comfort zone, to circumstances that aren't a sure thing. This, in fact, is the key to building confidence.

Most of us, however, don't gravitate toward such productive risk taking. We want guarantees of the "good life," and we've been trained to believe we can have it without experiencing any stress or struggle. Unfortunately, it's just not true. The best comedians, for example, are willing to dive headlong into the touchiest subjects and artfully restore our perspective where we have fallen into patterns of blind reactivity. Comedy teaches us to think sideways about ordinary life, to come at things from a fresh angle, and to step back and see ourselves and our challenging circumstances as though we were just bystanders watching the absurdity of our behavior, the folly of our seriousness. The comedian creates a bridge for his or her audience members, helping them to journey from their unconscious beliefs and reactions to conscious awareness and reflection.

Such perspective, provided by the comedian, is a form of mindfulness. We laugh because there is relief and delight when we gain a little distance from our reactive tendencies. In this way, comedians uplift us by leading us straight into the heart of our challenges.

> *I read this article. It said the typical symptoms of stress are eating too much, smoking too much, impulse buying and driving too fast. Are they kidding? This is my idea of a great day!* —Monica Piper

It's possible for anyone to develop a way to relate to stress that is much more self-aware, fun, and life-profitable.

If I asked you to name five primary sources of stress for yourself, you probably wouldn't have too much trouble coming up with a list. In fact, I invite you to try it. This will help get you into the spirit of the work we're going to do together here, which will involve your making a little effort if you want to handle your stress with more clarity. So go ahead and make a quick list of what you see as the root causes of your stress. (I'm waiting for you to actually do this…)

Okay, now have a look at your list and circle every item that is an *external cause*. Something that puts pressure on you as an outside force, like:

- My boss
- My children
- Money concerns
- Health issues
- Traffic

If you're like most people, your list of what seems to cause you stress falls into the category of *external conditions*. All of us face challenges that have real, practical, and logistical weight in our daily environments. The part we're not so practiced at seeing, however, is the extra stress-weight that we unconsciously add on top of those real challenges. So, yes, we have everyday problems and concerns that require us to make efforts to resolve them. However, I'm about to show you five extra layers of stress reaction that we *add* to the basic challenges of our lives. I call them *the secret stressors* because they remain mostly invisible to us unless we become practiced at noticing them. Each of the secret stressors is a confidence killer. The good news is that *we are the ones applying the stress*, which means we can stop!

Our ordinary life-challenges, before we dress them up in our own dire perspectives, are far more workable than we think. Not only that, but the organic stress of life is the grain of sand in the oyster of our success. Our challenges are the irritant we will build upon to grow our confidence.

Dave Scott is a six-time champion of the famed Ironman Triathlon. In terms of sporting events, it's an ultimate test, not just of physical endurance, but of mental fitness and attitude. This expert triathlete now teaches others how to train for the event. "I always ask people," he says, "'What do you want? And don't put any parameters on it.' Stress doesn't always have to be negative. I don't let people think too much about it. I tell them we're just going to do it. And quite often they do."[7]

Sage guidance from a peak performer who understands that we can't engage success when we're busy *reacting*, or letting ourselves "think too much" about our challenges. We must learn to *respond* to our stress with the appropriate mental attitude and the right action. And that involves making a distinction between the unadorned nature of our challenges and the stress reactions we bury ourselves under out of habit. Becoming aware of these reactions within us is how we stand a chance of responding effectively rather than behaving unconsciously when we're under pressure. When these stress reactions are not visible to us, we fight a losing battle, attempting to relieve ourselves as quickly as possible from the weight of stress without understanding how we are actually creating it. The act of seeking relief—and the quick fixes that seem to mitigate our stress in the moment—only compound the burden of our stress and amplify it in a downward spiral of stress reactivity.

The Downward Spiral of Stress Reactions

As I mentioned earlier, the disabling downward spiral of hidden stress begins with overt challenges.

- The potato doesn't cook.

- We get passed over again for a promotion we've been counting on.

- Our kid gets sick.

- A friend ignores us.

- We owe more tax than expected.

The unexpected twists and turns of daily life are guaranteed to keep coming at us.

In addition, there are challenges that excite us—the ones that arise from our heart of hearts as personal hopes and dreams. These are goals we aspire to, like deciding to participate in an Ironman competition, start a new business, or make a commitment to a life partner. Exciting opportunities and present potential can be just as stressful as negatively perceived events. But there's a common stress reaction that accompanies the moment when an external challenging issue, or an internal opportunity we're excited by, enters our attention.

We try to ignore it.

STRESS REACTION 1 — IGNORING REALITY

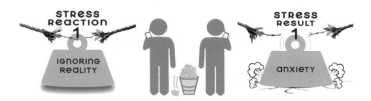

While awareness is how we rise to our best under pressure, ignorance is what keeps us down, unable to reach our highest hopes. *Ignore-ance is the act of pushing reality out of our attention.* The moment we register the presence of a challenge we're compelled to look away, distract ourselves, and avoid the issue. We're all guilty of this.

In our graphic for Stress Reaction One we see two individuals ignoring the piling up of trash. The trash needs to go out, but it's usually a thankless task (plus, why should *we* be the one who always has to do it?!). So we distract ourselves from the presence of the challenge by occupying our attention elsewhere.

Taking out the trash is, of course, a silly example, but not so silly when we consider the other simple activities we ignore and avoid to our disadvantage.

- Making an appointment to see the doctor or dentist
- Having a conversation with a colleague or friend about a way they've upset us
- Submitting a resume for a new job that could change our lives for the better
- Organizing our desk so we can do our best work

It's the ostrich method of stress management: putting our head in the proverbial sand and hoping that when we can't see our challenges they can't see us. Of course, that doesn't work.

Yes, sometimes ignored challenges will just go away on their own, yet often they only get worse in the absence of our attending to them. On the other hand, there is an objective weight to real challenges that can catalyze the brilliance of human responsiveness if we're willing to be present with them. That's what Dave Scott counts on when he encourages his trainees to embrace stress. Any challenging circumstance is an invitation for us to stretch our capacity and to engage creatively and adaptively with the situation. Like a kid who has no idea what the expected right answer is on a test but makes one up anyway. Such creative coping is a show of optimal human behavior. It is how children and adults alike can build their confidence and grow happier and more competent, each and every day.

Ignoring the presence of a challenge is a stress weight that we ourselves add which increases its force and overloads our capacity to manage it effectively. The stress result of *ignoring reality* is *anxiety*, which leaves us more uncomfortable than if we had just taken action. And, in an ironic twist, that anxiety triggers an even stronger effort to suppress the awareness of what we're feeling, which leads right into the trap of Stress Reaction Two and becomes a further assault on our confidence.

STRESS REACTION 2 — IGNORING EMOTIONS

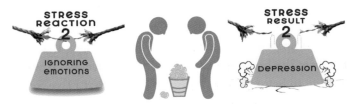

Recent neuroscientific study is now revealing complex links between memory, emotion, and decision making. These links are regulated by a part of the brain called the amygdala. When we push uncomfortable stimuli out of our attention, we're triggering a neurochemical process that—unattended by our awareness—can turn into a downward spiral of perception. Suppressing awareness of our inner *emotional states* can allow for a backfire of runaway activity in the amygdala. Such lack of awareness seems to play a pivotal role in allowing negative emotion to get the best of us. Something as relatively minor as taking out the trash becomes disproportionately distressing. Wanting to avoid this experience, we push feelings away with greater determination.

Feelings, unfortunately, cannot be selectively ignored. To cut off from feeling requires suppressing emotional energy on the whole. The result is depression. The disabling quality of depression neurologically scrambles our capacity for critical thinking, successful planning, and creative problem solving. We're then bathing our physical bodies in a stew of toxic tension. As we're pretending that our feelings are under control and report that we're "fine" when asked, our bodies bear the brunt of our unacknowledged suppression. "I never get angry," says Woody Allen. "I grow a tumor instead."

Also unfortunately, we are supported in the ignoring of our emotions by those who are presumed to have the most knowledge and authority. The medical establishment is a case in point. The link between stress and poor health has been ignored sufficiently in the past that in 2012 the American Psychological Association dedicated an entire research paper to the subject titled, "Stress in America: Missing the Healthcare Connection."

Dr. Gabor Maté is a bestselling author on the topics of addiction and stress. Regarding his own profession, he declares,

> *For all its triumphs and technical progress, mainstream Western medical practice militantly dismisses the role of emotions in the physiological functioning of the human organism. Its rejection of the mind/body unity is a classic case of denial.*[8]

Our feelings are a significant navigating force for action. When we distance ourselves from emotional intelligence by ignoring our feelings, we lose confidence in a primary source of our energy. In the process, we've set ourselves up to be at the effect of Stress Reaction Three, a stress which we have now manufactured for ourselves at a physiological level.

STRESS REACTION 3 — IGNORING PURPOSE

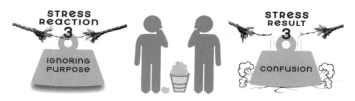

Having suppressed our emotions, we're left not knowing what we want or don't want, what we need or don't need, what we like or don't like, and we disconnect from our inner sense of direction and clarity in the moment. Increased activity in the amygdala clouds our judgment, overrides our sense of purpose, and causes us to forget our values. We start looking around, hoping to gain clues from the faces, behavior, or words of others. We defer to anyone who seems to have any authority or self-assurance. Yet others are no better prepared to lead with clarity than we are because they have been conditioned by the same cultural habits that have taken us all off course.

The question "Should we take out the trash or shouldn't we?" now becomes a major source of concern, prompting conversation, meetings, research, the taking of votes, and all manner of cogitation. And little of it produces results, because when no one has a clear feeling about things, there is no basis for confident action.

Such breakdown is highly detrimental to the functioning of corporate teams, families, sports teams, nonprofits, and political organizations and nations. Even if we don't belong to such groups or teams, we enact the conflict of procrastination, indecision, and overthinking *internally* among the many parts of ourselves that argue over what should be done next.

With the reaction of *ignoring purpose*, we've not only lost our personal clarity and agency, we're broadcasting our disorientation to the rest of our social environment, reinforcing the collective sense that nobody really knows what to do, and our sense of safety and confidence erodes in tandem with that of others. On our own, or with our teams, we then make poor decisions about our lives and the organizations we're meant to be serving. By this time, our limbic system is gearing up to intensify the amygdala's output of neurochemicals that are reserved for emergencies. This cocktail of stress-flammable juices starts to affect our thinking in ways that are dramatically absent of balanced perspective.

This panicked thinking becomes Stress Reaction Four, which, as you may have guessed, involves yet a further stage of ignoring the present truth and undermining our confidence.

STRESS REACTION 4 — IGNORING CREATIVITY

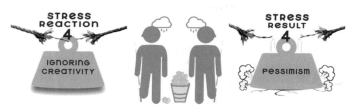

With this reaction, *ignoring creativity*, our brain function spirals further downward into a pit of negative thinking. Now we're assuming the worst, and best possible outcomes don't even occur to us. This is a type of reverse creativity, where we manufacture problems and ignore solutions. In scientific circles, this thought pattern that flares up under duress has a clinical name. It's called *negativity bias*.

Negativity bias produces a stockpile of cognitive distortions that causes us to overestimate and highlight problems, magnify the chances of catastrophe, and imagine the worst.

- If I put the trash out now, the wind could blow it over or animals might get into it. Then I'll have to clean up a bigger mess. I'll wait until tomorrow.

- It's already dark, and who knows who could be lurking in the alley?

- If I take out the garbage now, my boss might walk by and see my empty desk. He's already laid off two people this week. Better not give him a reason to think I'm slacking.

I've stuck to the trash analogy at the risk of trivializing just how neurologically dramatic negativity bias can be. For many, it has literally ended marriages, fueled crimes, and led to suicidal fantasies. We generate a stream of potentially terrible scenarios in this state—and because this biasing is all taking place unconsciously, we don't have the power to step in and regain balanced perspective or the capacity for reasonable action. We revert to any paths that haven't spelled disaster in the past, even if it means we doggedly commit to wholly unsatisfying situations.

If we were to step back and take an objective look at our reactivity, we might have a good laugh at the absurdity of our stress levels and our loss of confidence in relation to needing to take out the trash, make a simple phone call, ask our boss a question, or talk to our spouse about our feelings. Often, when we're reacting, a small amount of action at any point along the way can handle the matter and free us up to attend to the truly significant matters of our life. By the time we've triggered a negativity bias, however, we're quite embedded in our misperceptions and the lockdown that results.

The longer we stay stuck, the more we feed our collapse into this series of stress reactions. In the grip of our negativity bias, we don't question the exaggerated nature of our misperceptions. Instead, we defend them with logical sounding arguments and attempt to make our inaction seem like a reasonable choice. In truth, we are not seeing clearly when we're imagining the worst. Mark Twain sums it up nicely: "You can't depend on your eyes when your imagination is out of focus."

STRESS REACTION 5 — IGNORING ACTION

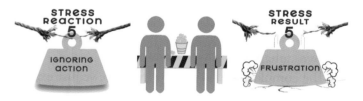

In this last stage of stress reaction, we defend our position with reasonable-sounding explanations for further inaction. We invent excuses and create obstacles to justify our lack of confidence. Rather than just saying, "I can't take out the trash because I panic at the thought of dark alleys," we say:

- "You know, I'm really not feeling well today."

- "My doctor advised me not to lift heavy things."

- "I believe this may contradict our policy. Let me have a look at the employee handbook and I'll get back to you tomorrow."

- "It's Sunday. Who takes the garbage out on a Sunday?"

Of course, at this point we haven't dealt in any material way with the simple issue at hand. Yet, internally we've created a highly charged, volatile state of fear and defense. In addition, our reactivity is out of our awareness and cloaked with justifications that we believe we have reasonable grounds for maintaining. We feel like a victim of our circumstance, deeply frustrated, without understanding how we have authored our own unhappy ending.

The cumulative effect of the cycle we've just examined compels us to try to escape feeling super stressed by ignoring issues more vigorously, which brings us back full circle to the beginning of the stress loop with a smaller sense of confidence in ourselves than ever.

Here's what the whole reactive stress-cycle looks like.

THE 5 STRESS REACTIONS & RESULTS

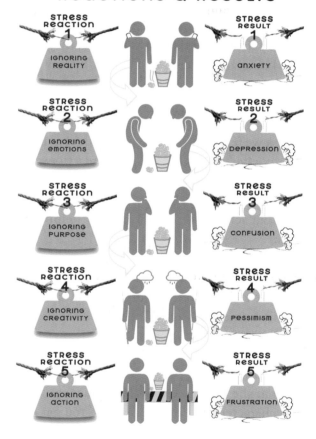

Now you have a sense of the stress reactions that were appropriate for helping us escape tigers in prehistoric times, yet in modern-day life trigger a downward spiral of unhappiness and dysfunction. These reactions feature very little reflective thinking. Yes, they do save us from being hit by cars and bitten by any snakes that might cross our path. The same neural pathways, unfortunately, are substantially less effective at helping us to hire a new employee, connect with our children when we're in a rush, or manage our money, time, and energy effectively. Our knee-jerk reactions do not serve us in contemporary adult life, where quick judgments based on a small amount of information, followed by big action, are not particularly helpful in the long run.

THE 5 STRESS REACTIONS IN DAILY LIFE

Perhaps the example of ignoring the pile up of trash doesn't hit home for you. Well then, imagine that a friend of yours, Karen, knows a business owner in an industry that you've dreamed of working in. Karen offers to introduce you. All you have to do is provide a resume that she can share as she puts in a strong word for your character and professionalism. You get excited and respond affirmatively when Karen asks if you want the introduction. "Great," she says. "Let me know when you have the resume." The ball is now completely in your court.

It's Monday morning. You tell yourself that it's the start of a busy week and it would be better to get a full workday in and then turn to resume writing. You decide you'll get the resume over to Karen first thing tomorrow. When tomorrow morning arrives, you realize that you forgot about a regular staff meeting you are obligated to attend, and you reschedule time to work on the resume in the afternoon. Once the afternoon rolls around, you feel exceptionally and unusually tired for some reason. You decide your best thinking is going to happen after a good night's sleep.

Reason after reason surfaces for delaying the writing and delivery of your resume. In truth, you're experiencing the first stress reaction, *Ignoring Reality*. In this case, you're ignoring the reality of a wonderful and positive opportunity. In his latest book, *The Big Leap*, Gay Hendricks identifies this form of reactivity as an "upper limit problem."[9] Mr. Hendricks's premise in this useful book is that we can experience stress not just when things go wrong, but when things go *right*.

Karen calls on Wednesday, wondering what's up. "You were so excited," she says, sounding a little confused. "By the way, I did mention to the business owner that you were interested in her company. She's totally excited to take a look at your background. But are you having second thoughts? Maybe you're feeling nervous about this?"

"No, not at all!" you declare, attempting to bury any awareness of your own waning confidence. "It's just been an unusually busy week. I'll get it over to you tomorrow."

Now you're denying your real feelings about the circumstance by *Ignoring Emotions*. What comes next is a sense of disorientation, because you've disconnected from the real direction in which your energy is moving or wants to go. Suddenly a feeling of being scattered and fragmented is casting a pall over everything you're supposed to be up to, disabling your ability to navigate to where you really want to go. Now you're *Ignoring Purpose*.

Next come the self-doubting thoughts, like, "I probably wouldn't get the job anyway. I'm really not qualified. What if I leave my job and this new one doesn't work out? That would be disastrous. What if I don't like the owner? That would put a big wedge between me and Karen." And the negativity doesn't stop there. It contaminates the rest of your current life circumstances, even without the prospect of the exciting, but stress-inducing, change. "I hate my job, I'll never get out of here, nothing ever works out for me," and on and on. You're now

Ignoring Creativity by allowing negativity bias to have a field day with your mind. The result is the illusory belief that you have no options and no hope. You are gripped by the convincing false impression that taking no action at all is actually the best thing to do in the moment, and that's just what you do, *Ignoring Action*.

This template repeats itself in the theater of our procrastination, even in relation to things we really want. Because it all occurs automatically and unconsciously, we end up feeling bewildered by the fact that we seem to function without confidence in our lives.

Now let's have a look at challenging interactions we have with our spouses, children, colleagues, neighbors, or friends. Perhaps you can recall a time when you were in the midst of a conversation and you noticed an expression of hurt or pain cross the face of the person you were speaking with. Did you ask what they were thinking? Did you inquire whether or not you said or did something that made them unhappy? Most of us shy away from opening up the can of worms that involves another person being unhappy with us. We'd rather let it blow over. When we ignore the hurt of another person, however, we're often just hurting ourselves by triggering the downward spiral of our own stress.

1. *Ignoring Reality*: The discomfort of someone finding fault with us is something we'd rather

not face if we don't have to. We'll attempt to ignore the upset of others if we suspect it involves them being critical of us.

2. *Ignoring Emotions*: When we sense we may be attacked, we bypass awareness of the fear that arises and go on attack before we realize what we're doing. (There are two forms our attacks typically take, depending on our personality type. In the first form, we start an argument, then blame or criticize the other person. In the second form, we become excessively hard on ourselves, harping on and exaggerating our own faults.)

3. *Ignoring Purpose*: Once our feelings get the better of us, they take on an overwhelming quality and short-circuit our clarity, distracting us from focusing on our present goals, like staying connected to our spouse, colleague, or friend.

4. *Ignoring Creativity*: Rather than problem solving with the individual or engaging in useful communication, we exaggerate the severity of the conflict and obsess over all the possible negative outcomes, ignoring the potential for positive resolution.

5. *Ignoring Action*: We come to the conclusion that it's much better to wait out the other

person's upset and hope it just goes away by itself than to wade into a conflict of unknown proportion. So we ignore the person or the issue altogether (which often just makes them more upset!).

Let's look at one more example of the downward spiral of stress reactivity. What about when we're the ones who feel wronged by somebody else? Imagine that you're working for a boss, manager, or supervisor who gives you occasional criticism and next to no positive feedback or guidance. How do you make this more stressful than it already is?

1. *Ignoring Reality*: You want to keep your job so you try to ignore the poor management environment you work within.

2. *Ignoring Emotions*: You're actually really mad at your boss, but you ignore your feelings, telling yourself and your colleagues (who think he's unprofessional) that it's not that bad.

3. *Ignoring Purpose*: You disconnect from the original enthusiasm and passion you initially had for your job and lose track of why you took the position in the first place.

4. *Ignoring Creativity*: You start to view your workplace, your role, and your boss in a highly critical

light that is greatly exaggerated in relation to your boss's occasional negative comments.

5. *Ignoring Action*: Finally, you stop making the efforts that produce great results, the habit of doing the bare minimum starts to creep into your routines, and you begin to actually get behind on deadlines and backed up on projects, which never happened before. Now you're actually delivering substandard results, which are totally out of character for you, and you begin to lose confidence in your abilities in the process.

This cycle we've been examining—layers of suppressed awareness that trigger a compound experience of self-created stress—is the breeding ground of neurosis. The word "neurosis" actually comes from the Greek word *neuron*, meaning "nerve." Paying attention to our nervous energy in a conscious manner helps us stem the tide of reaction. When we don't pay attention, our reactive habits wind up creating the very things we say we don't want. As Carl Jung said, "Neurosis is always a substitute for legitimate suffering." Legitimate suffering is the willingness to be with our pain and to allow our presence with it to guide our actions. This allows us to be responsive. In avoiding our pain, however, we wind up reacting. This also causes us suffering but we're creating much of it ourselves, as we've already discussed with regard to our habit of ignoring things.

Each of us has friends who come to us for support when challenges are present in their lives. When the suffering is "legitimate," we're all ears, and our empathy flows naturally alongside their sorrow and brings them comfort. When our friends are actually creating their own difficulties through avoidance strategies, yet claiming to be victims of circumstance, that same empathy is not elicited within us. Then we sit quietly thinking, "I feel like I've heard this before."

A SUMMARY OF THE FIVE STRESS REACTIONS

We have now set the stage for the story of our humanness—the story of how we've been trained to sell ourselves short on enjoyment and to perpetuate and protect our familiar and limiting experiences of stress. By way of summary, let's look through the lens of an ordinary circumstance, where a waiter doesn't live up to our expectations, to see what reactive habits actually look like and how we use them to buffer ourselves from intrusive feelings in challenging situations, yet make our stress worse and our confidence shakier in the process. I'm going to describe five reactive personality patterns that are fictional, but are based on common behavior I have seen in my actual training work with thousands of employees over many years.

IGNORING REALITY

Meet Phil, who arrived at one of my events with his wife, sat down, and immediately pulled out his phone to engage elsewhere. I couldn't help noticing his partner's disappointment, and I decided to try to help retrieve his attention. I started pouring water from behind them, as slowly as I could, just trickling it into the glass. I spent several minutes in this position, until the glass was finally completely full. His wife found the whole display hilarious, yet Phil never once looked up from his phone.

One of the first ways to deal with uncomfortable situations is to ignore them. We tune out and look for distractions. Cell phone and device use is rampant, obviously, and electronics provide a welcome diversion at events where large doses of human contact can leave us feeling exposed and anxious. The PEW Research Center recently found that 53 percent of people report having used their smartphone to avoid interacting with others, and 73 percent use their phone for no particular reason, just for something to do.[10]

Of course, the reality we're primarily avoiding is our feelings, particularly intrusive ones, and we haven't even begun to include the statistics about the other ways we avoid and ignore reality via our addictions, such as to entertainment, alcohol, work, and shopping. The result of such an avoidance habit is that our attention is easily captured by the flashiest, loudest, most sensational elements in any given environment. It's drawn from emergency to emergency, indulgence to indulgence, and distraction to distraction.

Because digital portals are everywhere, there are always sensationalized options available in any environment. We sleep, eat, and make love with our smartphones at arm's reach. As our attention is trained to prioritize ignoring our feelings using whatever distraction is available, our presence grows even weaker and the downward spiral of *ignoring* things begins, with reality receding into the background.

Phil's wife has repeatedly asked for his willingness to engage marriage counseling. After his refusing for several years, his wife informed him that she was ready to leave the relationship, after which he finally consented to giving counseling a try. Although they've been attending sessions for several months now, Phil has continued to declare that he doesn't see what the problem is with their marriage and that "everything is fine the way it is."

Denying that problems exist is a sure sign that we lack the confidence to engage them.

IGNORING FEELINGS

While watching me reach over the head of her col-league to pour water, Jill was experiencing strong negative feelings about the poor quality of my service. Unfortunately, there was no place in her world for those emotions. Rather than acknowledging them, she attempted to hide from her feelings and mask their presence from others by liter-ally covering her face with her hand. The word *persona* is Latin for "mask." The feelings that we allow or disallow in our lives form the personality mask we live behind. Cutting ourselves off from our feelings and masking any expression of them leaves us in a compromised position, because our inner life becomes unknown to us. In the absence of knowing for ourselves how we feel, we lose a primary form of navigating through our lives, and our potential for authentic expression becomes greatly diminished. Losing access to one's feelings in the midst of a challenge is like losing your map when you're trying to go to a place that you've never been. That's not a very confident position to journey from.

Jill is having some health problems that her doctor has told her are stress related. She is seeking a second opinion, as she feels sure it's purely a medical condition that is causing her sleep issues, even though 46 percent of women in America report they have trouble sleeping due to stress. Jill is always smiling and cheerful at work, despite constant stresses, like her explosive and belittling supervisor. Jill's friends have urged her to leave the company, but Jill maintains that it's not that bad.

IGNORING PURPOSE

Walking up behind Joe while he was seated at lunch, I began pouring water from quite a height above his head. I noticed him bend his head slightly forward as I trickled water into his glass. Just for fun, I lowered my arm a little bit. He responded by lowering his head some more. So I kept lowering my arm, thinking, "I wonder how far he'll go?" He actually bent forward so far beneath my lowering arm that he could have eaten his meal right off the plate without a fork. All the while that I enacted this bit of theater, he never questioned my actions: the point being that some of us are willing to bend over backwards (or forwards) in awkward situations to accommodate anyone who seems to be in charge, even if it's only a waiter.

In the absence of emotional awareness, we lack the inner guidance system we require to make clear decisions, speak up, say yes or no, sense the appropriateness of actions, or assess the wisdom of those who claim to be leaders. We become unsure of our own truth and default to following the crowd or those who are willing to be louder or more assertive.

Joe is constantly scrambling to keep his customers and meet their every need in the sales department of his company. Despite his efforts, his numbers are down. His VP wants Joe to negotiate with more backbone and stand for the value of the company and for his own time. Joe has been with the team for five years and is bewildered by why he keeps missing promotions as more junior recruits pass him by.

Ignoring Creativity

Karen wears a look of horror on her face that would be about right if she were witnessing an act of terrorism, yet is completely out of pro-portion to simply watching an individual overfilling a water glass. She is deeply worried about the behav-ior of her server and won-dering if he forgot to take his medication this morn-ing. Karen lives life in a state of mild-to-heightened panic, anticipating calamity and fearing the unknown. While the smallest departures from routine trigger her alarms, she stays ever watchful for potential threats.

As we become subconsciously aware that we are without internal strength and discrimination, we become fearful for our safety, and rightfully so. Without seeing it is within our power to address our fears through self-reflection, we project the cause of our fear onto the external environment and fall prey to negativity bias, the habit of imagining the worst in any given situation. We lose our confidence to a phantom army of potential disasters.

Karen is a stay-at-home mom who has already called her babysitter five times since she and her hus-band left the house to attend the event. Predictably, her kids tune her out as she attempts to keep them safe, clean, fed, and educated in a world she is sure will leave them dirty, ill, starving, and poorly prepared for the future if not for her constant intervention and "care."

IGNORING action

Ed is watching as I stretch across the entire banquet table where he is sitting. I'm trying to reach his glass to refill his water supply, and he's somehow content with watching me struggle to do it.

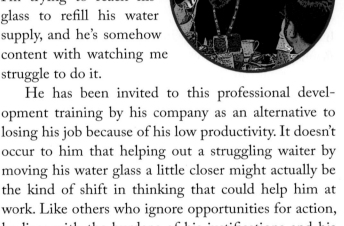

He has been invited to this professional development training by his company as an alternative to losing his job because of his low productivity. It doesn't occur to him that helping out a struggling waiter by moving his water glass a little closer might actually be the kind of shift in thinking that could help him at work. Like others who ignore opportunities for action, he lives with the burdens of his justifications and his logic—a thick layer of victim-*icing* on top of intrusive feelings—that keep him from believing his efforts can make any difference.

We all turn to the comfort of excuses, as they seem to promise a sense of reprieve from our stress. Indeed, excuses do provide a brief sense of relief, but underneath, every time we fail to take necessary action in our lives, we become less confident in our capacity to cope with our challenges.

About a year ago, Ed suffered a mild heart attack. He has assured his family and boss that exercise will become a priority for him, though he hasn't yet found the opportunity to rearrange his busy schedule to fit it in.

How can we better handle our stress?

In the opening statements of her book *Better Than Before*, author Gretchen Rubin reports, "We repeat about 40 percent of our behavior almost daily."

We are indeed "creatures of habit," and once these behavioral grooves are established, the decisions we make, even in critical circumstances, will fall in line with the physiological momentum of those habits, which are embedded in our cells, sinews, muscles, bone and nerves. As we've discussed, this makes us more prone to reacting than it does to optimally responding. The important thing about habits is that we be aware of them and that we review them on a regular basis, assessing whether they are supportive of our true wishes, our sense of purpose, and our direction in life. If they are, we can choose to maintain them. If our habits are actually reaction based and not supportive of our current real wishes, we can practice letting them go and find new behaviors that better suit our goals and intentions.

What we've covered so far in this section of the book is how, by default, we behave in alignment with a set of reactive habits that are

- not in our awareness.

- not freely chosen.

- not supportive of living our best lives.

Reactive habits defend us from intrusive feelings, make the stresses of our lives worse, and stop us from proceeding with clarity, creativity, and confidence.

Let's assume that we've now become convinced that ignoring

- reality

- emotions

- purpose

- creativity and

- action

is not a good idea. So how do we turn this habit around? How can we stop ourselves from being drawn into a downward spiral of stress? Even better, how can we actually build our confidence under pressure and turn stress to our advantage? That will be our focus in Part Two.

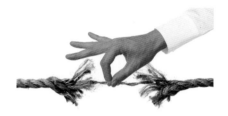

PART TWO

HOW TO
CONFIDENTLY TAKE
CHARGE OF YOUR STRESS

5 QUESTIONS FOR CONFIDENTLY TAKING CHARGE OF STRESS

In Part One we've had an in-depth look at what really causes stress and how we make our stress worse than it needs to be with our unconscious reactions to life's challenges. This book addresses the opportunity we have to reverse those reactive patterns and to handle our stress in a productive, rather than unconscious, manner. New habits, however, take time to build and reinforce. Perhaps you're stressed right now and need an immediate solution for your pain. If you aren't feeling stressed at the moment, there's a reasonable chance you might be before the day is out.

Here, in Part Two, I'm going to introduce you to a set of tools that will be immediately helpful for taking charge of your stress. The tools all happen to be questions. Questions are a powerful form of leverage when it comes to directing our attention, decisions, and actions. David Hoffeld, the author of *The Science of Selling*, explains the power of questions.

> *So why do questions have such influence on the decision-making process? First and foremost, they prompt the brain to contemplate a behavior, which increases the probability that it will be acted upon. In fact, decades of research has found that the more the brain contemplates a behavior, the more*

likely it is that we will engage in it. That's not all. Just thinking about doing something can shift your perception and even alter your body chemistry.[1]

The questions I am about to share with you have been specifically designed to lead your brain down a new neural pathway when under stress. The questions will help you to "sell" yourself on an alternative way of perceiving and acting when the pressure is on. That new perception will, in turn, build the degree of confidence you have when approaching stressful circumstances.

CONFIDENCE BUILDING QUESTION 1 – WHAT AM I IGNORING?

Earlier, we examined the stress reactions and associated stress results that deepen our sense of anxiety and our chance of getting stuck in relation to our challenges. Now we're going to look again at the same five stress points and explore five confidence building questions we can apply under those conditions to better respond to our stress.

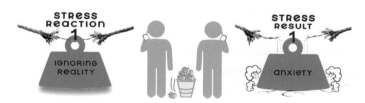

The first stress reaction we've already discussed in Part One is *Ignoring Reality*, resulting in anxiety. Unconsciously, we often push the things that make us uncomfortable out of our attention. Or, alternatively, we may distract ourselves entirely from the situation at hand.

Presence is the fundamental competency that allows us to handle stress with confidence. As a means of restoring presence in a challenging circumstance, we can use the question, "What am I ignoring?"

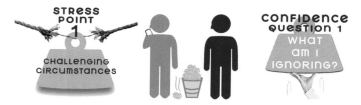

The ability to notice what we've pushed into the background of our awareness and to remain calmly alert in any given environment is a very necessary skill. This is the first step toward restoring balance neurologically, taking charge of our stress and positioning ourselves to respond usefully to a challenge at hand.

Tarini Bauliya is a corporate sales consultant and a former sales executive for Proctor and Gamble. She attributes her success with organizational sales teams to a method of *embracing the present moment*. Here's how she described it in my recent interview with her.

Frequently, a customer in a sales exchange says something we don't want to hear. They throw something from left field at us. The tendency is to seek out more familiar and comfortable territory. Unconsciously, we're thinking, "I don't want to hear this." We don't allow new information in because it doesn't allow us to stay on course with our script—it throws us for a loop. When we try to avoid that [discomfort of the unfamiliar] rather than follow it, we shut down possibility. In actuality, when that thing comes from left field, it's coming from a field of opportunity. In a sales setting, that's the very thing I like to invoke.

Asking ourselves "What am I ignoring?" can serve as a gentle reminder to allow the *field of opportunity* to reveal itself to us. The trick is to approach the question with an open mind, unoccupied by preconceptions about what the answer should be.

We all become quite skilled at setting up our lives in a way that helps us to steer around our *stress triggers*. Consciously applied, this strategy can be a useful form of stress management; however, when our stress triggers are active, we tend to react by abandoning the journey altogether. In the process, we've unconsciously sabotaged the scope of our life engagement. The practice is to let our subconscious—or we could even say "to let our body"—speak its wisdom. It works best if we don't overthink what arises when we ask the question "What am I ignoring?," even if the answer that comes to us doesn't make immediate sense.

If you're game to give it a try now, you might make a short list of what pops into your mind when you ask yourself, "What am I ignoring?" It could be anything that needs attention: an email you've delayed replying to, a messy desk, a dirty bathroom. It could be an object, a circumstance, a part of town, a person, an opportunity, a phone call or conversation, an errand. The seemingly smallest things can get unconsciously pushed into the background of our attention in an attempt to avoid our stress triggers.

Directing this question, "What am I ignoring?" *internally* is equally valid and useful. We could look at this question as a modulating wave of presence, where we ask what might need our attention in the *outside* world, as well as what could use our attention *inside* of ourselves.

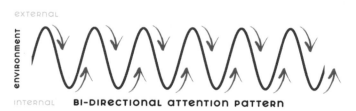

BI-DIRECTIONAL ATTENTION PATTERN

By directing our attention toward the details of our daily lives and discerning what we might be ignoring—and alternately directing our awareness toward our inner condition—we create an effective net for detecting root sources of stress. This openness and fluidity of attention is the cornerstone of developing confidence in ourselves. We need to become reliably present to the reality of our lives.

In a given moment, we might feel as though there is nothing we are ignoring in our outer environment. When we look inside ourselves, however, and find that our stomach is churning, our shoulders are tense, or our jaw is clenched, we have a useful starting point for taking charge of our stress rather than being blindsided by it later on.

On the other hand, we may not be completely tuned in to our internal state, but we might notice that the thought of attending a particular meeting fills us with dread. Externally perceived stresses can be a reminder to track our inner reactions and the way they show up physiologically. We might find a sinking feeling in the pit of our stomach, heaviness in our chest, or other corresponding manifestations of internal stress.

Whether we start outside or inside, our experience of being stressed *always* includes a physical component. It could be a physical ache or pain, tension somewhere in the body, or some other discomforting sensation. Such sensations might show up as variations of temperature, pressure, or pain: hot, sweaty, damp, chilled, heavy, pressing, constricting, pinching, aching, poking, cramping. There are multitudes of sensations that we may not even consciously register from moment to moment, but when it comes to moving past moderately imprinted forms of trauma, awareness of disquieting sensations in the body is essential. It is being aware of these sensations *in advance of our reactivity to them* that allows us to choose an alternative response.

Awareness of our sensations makes it possible to dissolve habitual fixations we have on old and ineffective methods of coping with stress. That's what reactions are: unconscious fixations on solutions that don't work. Those fixations can only sustain themselves where there is physiological denial. We *re*-act, again and again, until we can accept our experience fully. The biological self seeks to resolve stressful episodes by opening to the full measure of the trauma's impact. If we block, suppress, and ignore the feeling-sensations associated with these past events, the trauma will only surface again and again until we've fully acknowledged those feelings.

Dr. Peter Levine is a foremost researcher on the subject of stress and trauma. Thirty years of study and therapeutic practice are distilled in his widely acclaimed publications on the subjects. In his book *Waking the Tiger*, Dr. Levine tells us, "The healing of trauma is a natural process that can be accessed through an inner awareness of the body.[2] Healing trauma requires a direct experience of the living, feeling, knowing organism."[3]

Asking ourselves what needs our attention and openly scanning our external and internal environment is the first step of our awareness journey. That awareness allows us to identify where our greatest sources of energy are hidden. When we're in denial of any energetic knots in our inner or outer field, our vitality becomes bound and is unavailable for use toward conscious aims. Developing confidence to handle stress requires that we locate those energy sources as a first step. This turns a field of hidden obstacles into what Tarini Bauliya, quoted above, calls a "field of opportunity."

While pushing things out of our attention is one way in which we *ignore reality*, another misuse of our attention is to overanalyze a present challenge, obsess over it, put it under a microscope, and "miss the forest for the trees," as the saying goes.

It may be difficult to see how we are ignoring reality when all of our attention seems to be laser-focused on coping with a stress. Much of our stress, however, is characterized by excessive rumination on a limited area of concern. The natural consequence is that we ignore the broader context of our lives.

Perhaps we have financial challenges, and as we work ourselves into a knot of panic and despair we don't notice that we're sitting on our front porch in the sun, the birds are singing, the sun is setting, and we're in good health. We easily forget that there is no life-threatening emergency in the moment when we're triggered by a stress reaction.

In addition to the question "What am I ignoring?," any form of inquiry that helps us reorient to the here and now can be useful, such as,

Where am I?

What task am I in the middle of?

What are my immediate surroundings?

It's true that stress can wreak havoc with our lives, and habitual stress, especially over long periods, can leave us physiologically damaged and chemically imbalanced. For many of us, our stress levels are not quite that entrenched. But whether our anxiety level has us balled up and cowering in a corner or just mildly distracted in the moment, *the first step toward managing stress right now is to stabilize our presence. Every additional competency we need for taking charge of our stress requires our steady presence as a foundation.*

CONFIDENCE BUILDING QUESTION 2 – WHAT AM I FEELING?

Once we've become consciously aware of what we've been avoiding, we're likely to have some strong feelings about it, since underlying uncomfortable feelings are what cause us to turn away from stressors in the first place. If we're reacting by *Ignoring Emotions*, we can deepen our anxiety to the point of depression.

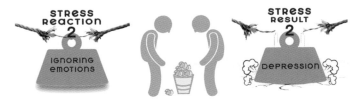

To reverse the reactive cycle at this point, we turn to Confidence Building Question 2, which is "What am I feeling?"

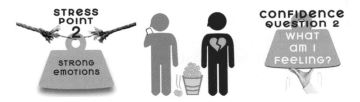

Returning to the overflowing trash example, we might answer, "I'm really sad that nobody else cares about keeping this place clean."

In Part One, I shared some of the neuroscience behind emotional suppression and how our limbic system can become overstimulated, resulting in runaway activity of the amygdala. This disables the prefrontal cortex, to which we need stable access if we wish to be at our best under pressure. *Feeling* is a source of fuel for action—until it overtakes our capacity to integrate it. When feelings are having *us* instead of us having *them*, the information we get from feeling can't be imported into clear thinking, useful decision making, and optimal action.

Numerous studies have shown that we can easily increase, rather than repress, the awareness of our emotions just by naming them.[4] Obviously, there are many nuances of feeling, and as we initially experiment with labeling them, it's best to keep the options simple. Even among leading psychologists in research and practice there is some debate about our basic human emotions, yet a good number of independent theorists have suggested the universality of six feeling states.[5]

- Happiness

- Surprise

- Fear

- Sadness

- Anger

- Disgust (combined with contempt)

When feeling stressed, we might choose to review an even shorter list, inquiring as to whether we're feeling…

- Mad
- Sad
- Scared or
- Bad

…to provide ourselves with a quick anchor for neurochemical stability. Specifically, labeling our emotions can activate the ventrolateral prefrontal cortex and reduce emotional amygdala reactivity.

Feelings, however, are a seductive subject when it comes to our attention. Reflecting on his clinical experience, Dr. Levine reports that

because emotions can be powerful, compelling, dramatic, and intriguing, they present a special challenge for working with the felt sense. Most people find emotions a far more interesting topic of investigation than mere sensations. However, if you want to learn to use the felt sense, and especially if you want to learn to use the felt sense to resolve trauma, you must learn how to recognize the physiological manifestations (sensations) that underlie your emotional reactions.[6]

As we put our attention on our feelings with the hope of naming them, we may find ourselves getting swept away by their dramatic power. We may be drawn into habitually negative patterns of thought and even counterproductive actions that don't serve us when we're under the influence of emotional intensity.

In her book *Emotional Agility,* psychologist Susan David describes two ineffective ways of processing emotion, which she calls "bottling" and "brooding."

The one is ignoring emotions; the other is dwelling on emotions. Yet both are interestingly associated with lower levels of ability to deal with stress, to be productive and to solve problems.[7]

To transform the stress of both bottling and brooding, we'll do well to remember that our experience of any given emotion is actually a collection of sensations. If we have difficulty finding clarity in the midst of an emotional whirlwind, we can turn to naming *sensations.* "What am I feeling *in the body*?" is a modification of the question that can help us to reorient, using some of the tools for presence we've already discussed. From there, we can bridge back to naming feelings in a more general manner. Without the capacity for presence and a grounded relationship to the present moment, asking ourselves what we're feeling can be a setup for feeling overwhelmed by our experience.

Science has shown that simply giving our feelings a name really helps, *once we are reasonably anchored in the present*.[8] By naming them, we become more confident in our ability to relate to our feelings and emotions in a useful way. The benefits of this step will become even clearer as we move to question three.

CONFIDENCE BUILDING QUESTION 3 – WHAT AM I REALLY WANTING?

The third reaction to stress is *Ignoring Purpose*, which leads to a sense of confusion.

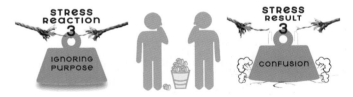

Now, however, in the flow of our confidence building questions, we're already well on our way to bypassing a confused state. The awareness process we establish with the first two questions opens our attention, balances our perception, and gives us increased access to the kind of objective experiencing that is assisted by the prefrontal cortex. The questions help us to collect our attention and identify the emotions that are present for us in relation to stressors. This puts our emotions in context and balances our perspective. With Question 3, we're going to take advantage of that perspective and ask ourselves "What am I really wanting?"

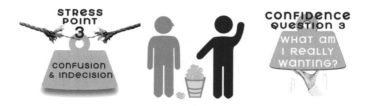

We're now in a position to identify or name what we want without being wholly identified with whatever emotional charge may be present, and to consider our own broader life experience, goals, and heartfelt wishes, as well as the factors of our current environment and the people we're sharing that environment with. Without dismissing our present feelings, we can make decisions that reflect the full measure of our wisdom and presence. This disposition is the ground of what some might call having a "vision," either for this moment or for the long-term future of our lives. The question "What am I really wanting?" can provide us with useful direction. In the same way that labeling emotions calms the amygdala, identifying a focus for ourselves, even if it's not permanent or perfect, has the further effect of optimizing our neurochemistry.

Sometimes it is not immediately possible to identify what we want. We may need to hold this question lightly as we move forward with whatever work or tasks are currently before us. If we can hold the question, we will often find ourselves delighted or surprised by the answer that eventually comes to us. Strangely, developing awareness of our personal feelings and wishes often puts us in touch with aspirations that are beyond a personal frame. The perspective provided by this question may naturally lead to altruistic visions and an inspiration to serve greater causes. What we're doing is opening ourselves to a broader *field* of awareness that some people claim is key to entering a flow state; others even equate it with spiritual experience. This could simply feel like a sense of knowing what is needed around us—a feeling of what the right thing to do is, even if it doesn't match our personal life script or immediate individual concerns. The obviousness of what is wanted and needed in the moment may override our personal agenda. The question "What am I really wanting?" can open us to what *reality itself* is really wanting. It's not that our personal sphere is irrelevant to this broader perspective. Our personal experience becomes a factor held in a larger context rather than becoming the gravitational center of our attention, which is the cause of reactive behavior.

Using this process over time, you will likely reveal "wants" that run the gamut from ordinary personal requirements, like "I want a nap," to universal and grand visions like "I want all children in this world to live without hunger." Natural evidence of this process often shows up in the work of artists who respond to the call of creative action, which allows them to produce something that seems to come from beyond themselves.

We don't need to judge the mundane aspects of personal need when they're present, or expect that we should always be pursuing global visions. We can just let this questioning process reveal what is naturally there for us moment to moment. As we become more practiced at remaining connected to a bigger picture, even when under stress, we begin to trust our ability to maintain clarity in the face of our challenges. Once again, we're growing our confidence in general while immediately restoring perspective.

CONFIDENCE BUILDING QUESTION 4 – WHAT'S A USEFUL BELIEF?

Anytime we identify what we want, we activate our imagination and begin to contemplate how our wish could come true. Simultaneously, however, declaring a vision for ourselves can trigger a human tendency we'll want to pay attention to, which is called *negativity bias*. We've previously discussed the effects of negativity bias in Part One. Briefly, it's an error of human perception where we give more weight to negative events, comments, interactions, and outcomes than we do to those that are positive.

Do you believe that imagination is a wonderful thing? If you're like most people, you'll say yes. And it is, except for the 90 percent of the time we use it to imagine the worst. Could this have been what the creative genius Walt Disney was referring to when he declared, "I resent the limitations of my own imagination"? Negativity bias leads us to imagine the worst before we envision the best, especially when we find ourselves in already stressful circumstances.

This describes the fourth stress reaction, *Ignoring Creativity*, which we've previously examined. Ignoring our capacity for intentional creativity allows negativity to take over. Technically, I guess we'd have to say that extreme negativity *is* a form of creativity. Creativity that takes the form of a useful belief, however, sets the stage for positive change.

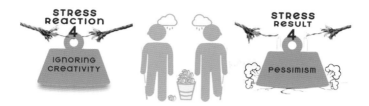

We've already done ourselves a favor by using the first three questions to connect to the strength of conscious presence (What needs my attention?), emotional awareness (What am I feeling?), and declared intent (What am I really wanting?). Those questions are a powerful force. If we hold them in mind as we look for ways to move forward, we'll start giving more weight to our possibility for success and less gravity to the consequences of a potential failure.

The fourth confidence building question, "What's a useful belief?," works in beautiful partnership with the others. A *useful belief* is simply the counterbalance to negativity bias. A *useful belief* helps us to see the possibilities that exist in the present moment.

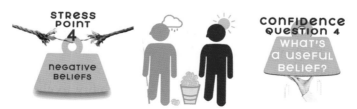

If it's a cloudy day, thinking that it will probably rain on us if we take out the trash right now is an example of negativity bias. Thinking that the sun might come out is a useful belief. Not because it's certainly true, but because it's a belief that invites us forward into our lives. Even if we're not able to visualize a sunny future, just reminding ourselves that we can handle a little rain if it happens to occur is a useful belief.

Speaker and author Chris Helder wrote the book on *Useful Belief*, literally. He explains it like this:

> *Let's say you walk into that meeting you can't avoid with a different attitude. You decide to adopt a useful belief about the meeting. You are confident that something productive will come of it, or that you will learn something or encounter some new ideas. Notice what happens then. Your reticular activating system will search for something useful to come out of the meeting. Maybe something useful will be there, maybe it won't. Either way, if it is there, you will find it.*[9]

Said even more simply, in the words of American philosopher and psychologist William James, "The greatest weapon against stress is our ability to choose one thought over another."

When I shared this useful belief concept with one man, he expressed his concern that he'd be lying to himself using this method, leading himself into a false sense of confidence in his circumstances or abilities. A useful belief, I told him, has three requirements:

1. It is formulated only after we have stopped ignoring reality, our emotions, and our most heartfelt desires.

2. It declares openness to a new potential.

3. Our desire to see if it's true inspires immediate action.

A useful belief is not a fantasy; rather, it's a kind of costume we put on to play with possibility. We're not blinding ourselves to our past experience or putting ourselves naively in danger by ignoring everything we've learned so far in life. What we're doing is counterbalancing negativity bias by rediscovering our childlike optimism, when we practiced starting sentences in our mind with the words "What if…" and completed them with best-case scenarios.

The most successful innovators, leaders, and problem solvers see a world different from the one you or I do when they look at a challenging circumstance. That difference comes from the practice of suspending what we *know* in order to open ourselves to what *might be*.

Useful beliefs remind us of the capacity, options, and choices that we always have as we approach even stressful circumstances. In short, a useful belief will lead us toward a useful action. Gaining some mastery over which beliefs we use to build our future is a big step toward living more confidently.

CONFIDENCE BUILDING QUESTION 5 – WHAT STEP CAN I TAKE?

If we've actually identified a useful belief for ourselves, we will be naturally motivated to move into action. We are well positioned to avoid the trap of *ignoring action* that is part of the reaction cycle we've been studying.

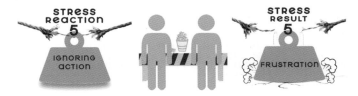

The difficulty we can fall into here is trying to do too much at once. If we see a big challenge as something we need to conquer all at once, it's likely we'll continuously delay the process of addressing it. The question "What step can I take?" prompts us to identify one small step we can take right away to get moving in the right direction.

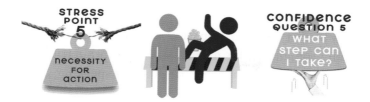

STRESS
POINT
5

necessity
FOR
action

CONFIDENCE
QUESTION 5
WHAT
STEP CAN
I TAKE?

When we're under stress, we can come up against what is called the *freezing response*, where the simplest action, for some inexplicable reason, becomes difficult or impossible for us to take. Most of us have experienced this, where the smallest task fills us with a kind of dread. In stressful circumstances, we'll want to work with micro-steps that get us moving in the right direction and are minor enough that they don't trigger a freezing response. Once we're in motion, we're less likely to become a victim of such paralysis.

If taking out the trash is the goal, or what we're really wanting, it helps to make a distinction between our ultimate destination and the steps along the way. So, here, the next step could just be, "I can pick up the trash bin." We handle one hurdle at a time in small doses, and this keeps us moving forward in action. Under stress, our steps need to be small. Once we've identified what we're really wanting, we simply look for small, easily performed bridging actions that will naturally lead us in the direction of our larger goal.

As a final note about making an effort, I suggest it may be that the small step we embrace is to *refrain* from doing something. It's a small step to stop interrupting your spouse for a day when he or she is speaking, or to hold your tongue when you'd usually put yourself down after being complimented, or to refrain from having the extra drink before leaving the bar. In fact, what we *stop* doing, in small conscious increments, can be every bit as life changing as what we *start* doing.

THE 5 CONFIDENCE BUILDING QUESTIONS IN REAL LIFE

The five questions I've outlined are natural anchors for confidence that we instinctually gravitate toward as human beings. Once again, we see such naturalness in the behavior of children. I recently took my son up a chairlift in the mountains of Park City, Utah, to enjoy the summer recreational activities. The ride up was beautiful, but it was a chairlift, exposed to the elements, drifting high above the ground as it silently elevated us thousands of feet up the lush-green, snowless ski run. The stress of the circumstance in the eyes of my child came from his perception of our vulnerability, suspended up there in space. He didn't try to divert his attention away from the circumstance, however. Instead, he naturally behaved in a way that helped him to turn his stress around.

1. He didn't try to ignore what was alarming to him, which allowed him to stay present in the experience of his concern.

2. He turned to me and said, "Daddy, I'm scared," naming his feeling.

3. Then he asked, "They have a way of getting us down from here if it stops, right, Dad?," indicating that what he really wanted was reassurance.

4. Before I could even answer his question, he turned his imagination toward creating a small army of useful beliefs. He started with "I'll bet they have something like helicopters waiting in case people get stuck." "Yes," I said, "or maybe some big air bags they inflate that we could jump into." His eyes lit up as he started imagining all the different ways we might be rescued, like "Maybe they have a million marshmallows and they spread them all out into a big pile!" We spent a few minutes exchanging wildly creative ideas about how we could get down safely, until he concluded, "They probably have some really good ways of getting people down we haven't even thought of."

5. These stress-reversing perceptions set him up for simple, practical action. He scooted right

over close to me and said, "Dad, can you hold onto me?," which I did, and he freely enjoyed the rest of the ride.

In children, we can see the natural process of stress-surfing in action. It's actually not complicated or foreign to natural human behavior. It's a form of common sense that unfortunately becomes uncommon as unresolved trauma locks us into stress precedents that disconnect us from responsiveness.

What might the natural unfolding of confident questioning look like in an excelling organization, as practiced by a leader? In an interview I recently had with Denny's CEO John Miller, he recalled a story about one of his most important mentors, Norman Brinker. Mr. Brinker created the Brinker International hospitality empire that gave rise to the success of the Chili's, Macaroni Grill and other concepts decades ago, and John Miller considered himself privileged to have been mentored by him.

Miller's story involved an incident where a restaurant employee was alone late one night, closing shop in one of the locations, when someone knocked loudly on the service entrance claiming to be in need of help and begging to be let in. Store policy is strict on the matter. Under no conditions is an employee to open the doors to a restaurant after closing time. The visitor was convincing enough, however, to compel the employee to open the door. The staff member immediately found himself being held up at gunpoint for the contents of the store register.

John Miller recounted the conversation among the leadership team that occurred the next day at the regional managers' staff meeting. It just so happened that the meeting was being attended by Norman Brinker himself. The rank and file was swift and decisive in the need to terminate the employee, perhaps even more resolute to follow the rules in the presence of their founder. Brinker, however, interrupted with a question, asking, "Why would you want to do that?"

The room went silent as someone tentatively offered, "Because that's our policy. He broke the rules, and look what happened."

"Yes," Brinker agreed. "But what are the chances that this employee will ever do that again?"

A unanimous "no chance at all" was the response, and Brinker explained his reasoning for keeping the employee on staff. "What you need to do," he said, "is make this young man the spokesperson for this policy. Empower him to set the example of why we abide by this rule."

"No one in the room could argue with the logic of the approach," John Miller noted. In addition, as was clearly the case for Miller, those attending were inspired by the application of transformative thinking in a stressful circumstance.

Clearly, Brinker hadn't heard of my five-question method for turning stress around. The truth is that these five questions represent the energetic disposition of natural authority that we see active in the behavior of exceptional leaders. Here's how I imagine Norman Brinker might have answered our five questions if he'd been asked that day.

1. *What am I ignoring?* The future life of an employee.

2. *What am I feeling?* Compassion for someone who made a big mistake.

3. *What am I really wanting?* This employee to succeed and our company to thrive.

4. *What's a useful belief?* Mistakes afford the greatest learning, which makes this employee a valued member of our organization.

5. *What step can I take?* Give him the opportunity to make amends and to flourish as a leader from the seed of experience.

We might typify the context of leadership as *the ability to hold stress as an opportunity rather than as an obstacle to be quickly eradicated.* Moving *toward* stressful circumstances rather than avoiding them requires that we sacrifice the habit of our quick judgments and low tolerance for risk. Such a capacity inspires confidence in both the leader and those he or she is leading.

Father Daniel Joseph Berrigan was a Jesuit priest who led a series of antiwar protests, especially during the years of the U.S. war in Vietnam. In a recent interview, Martin Sheen recalled being arrested alongside Father Berrigan in a 1986 protest.[10] Referring to the strength of Father Berrigan's beliefs, Sheen comments, "If what we believe doesn't cost us something, then we are left to question its value." He was referring in this context to Father Berrigan's willingness to go to jail.

Ironically, when it comes to living with greater confidence, the sacrifice we have to make is to step *out of jail*, leaving the prison of our old reactions behind. We sacrifice the familiar cell of our confining past, the comfort of established routines, the safety of policy, and our old ideas about how large a challenge we can handle.

A few months ago I was due to leave for a business trip early on a Monday morning. It would be a long day and I needed a good night's sleep. I had been reading some literature on climate change, including Naomi Klein's latest book, *This Changes Everything*.[11] Despite the book's thoughtful and inspired approach to addressing a substantial planetary stress, my own mind had cantered out into a minefield of alarmist scenarios. In a state of reclined panic, I just couldn't sleep. I felt overwhelmed by the magnitude of our global climate challenge. I really needed to get some rest, and my first reaction was to try to ignore the whole thing. Needless to say, that didn't work.

I was already writing this book, and I'd spent a good hour lying awake in the middle of the night before it occurred to me to apply what I'd been describing as the answer to stress!

So I went through the questions.

1. *What am I ignoring?* The reality of climate change.

2. *What am I feeling?* Scared about what will happen to the planet, mad that most of us are ignoring the issue, sad that I'm part of the problem and have to take a car to the airport tomorrow to get on a plane, both of which are going to contribute to the very thing I feel upset about.

3. *What am I really wanting?* To at least do my part not to unnecessarily add to the problem.

4. *What's a useful belief?* I can find some way to lessen the impact of my travel by finding alternatives.

5. *What step can I take?* Shamefully, I hadn't been a public transit person, so my first thought was to check out the bus schedule. I discovered the buses didn't run as early as I needed to leave, but just the act of getting up and actually checking for transit options shifted something inside of me. Just taking that small action felt so good that it turned on my sense of agency. It was then that I had a truly radical idea. I could bike to the airport.

Although this idea was exciting to me, it brought yet another opportunity to work with the fearful projections of my own mind. I knew I'd be riding in the dark, there was potential for rain, and I'd be riding on roads not designed for cyclists. I watched my mind sliding into its penchant for negativity, thinking it would be too far, too early in the morning, too wet, too dangerous. Then I started imagining myself missing my plane or, worse, winding up in the hospital from a road accident. But I followed through and challenged all the stress precedents that were internally triggered by the commitment to bike rather than drive.

In the end, I woke early enough to load up my bike, make the ride, and arrive at the airport on time. I was able to use some bike carriers and a backpack to bring everything I needed for the trip, and I found a bike rack at the airport, where I locked my bike. In reality, it turned out to be no big deal. It was a vivid and remarkable example of how convincing our imagined limits can appear when we're in the grip of fear. Breaking through the barrier of my own old habits gave me an enormous amount of energy that stayed with me for the whole trip, despite the short night's sleep and the extra physical effort required. Upon my return, I rode home not only without incident, but eliminating a small amount of carbon pollution, saving gas, and, most important, filling my own inner fuel tank with a massive sense of capacity and agency.

Laziness is not the simple vice we often label ourselves or others with. It's a euphemism for a complex weave of stress reactions that disable us from doing the optimal thing in a given moment. In short, the real climate tragedy is *inside of us*. It's our *inner* climate that is out of whack, devoid of the confidence we need to take effective and useful action. No surprise then that our outer climate suffers from our inflexibility— just as a family suffers when parents refuse to address their own reactivity, and any organization suffers when leaders enforce rigid adherence to rules and policies that are more about staying in control than about achieving a mission.

If we really want to address global warming, we have to attend to the confidence cooling that we've fallen prey to through our modern-day habits of inattentiveness, fear-based reactivity, and action paralysis. Could global warming, along with a host of other large-scale stresses, be a symptom of the human spirit misfiring? I believe that it's the personal transformation of thought, mood, and action that positions us usefully in relation to our current lives and the needs of our families, jobs, community, and world. If we keep ourselves in useful motion, enthusiastically applying our life force to our highest wishes from moment to moment, challenging the creep of our shrinking limits, we will live our best lives, and the world will get the best we have to offer.

Whether or not any of our small efforts make a difference in a given circumstance is irrelevant. Riding my bike to the airport obviously didn't solve the climate crisis, but it immediately addressed my personal confidence crisis and allowed me to respond to my stress in a useful manner.

These questions will become more effective as you practice them over time. But, make no mistake, our old habit patterns are deep, and it takes effort and work to build new pathways to a confidence-rich life. Upon first application you may find that answers to the five questions are not always obvious, despite their simplicity. In the beginning stages we're likely to feel that this questioning process doesn't work for us, that we're actually not ignoring anything, that we're feeling nothing, that we don't know what we want or even believe that anything different is possible. Even if these questions and the answers they generate initially feel ineffective or inaccessible, I guarantee that if you're willing to practice drawing upon them when the pressure is on, they will start giving you a much greater sense of confidence for handling your life challenges. I recommend you begin by applying the questions to mild stressors until you get used to working with them. This will eventually prepare you to use them effectively even in much more dramatic situations.

As you become more skilled at navigating the labyrinth of your old reactions, you'll come to see how natural and easeful it is to respond to these five invitations for increased awareness. If you get stuck in the learning process, you can even skip a question in the sequence, insert answers that make you laugh, ask a friend for help, put the process away and come back later fresh.

Start where you are, move where you can, and keep using these questions to bring a natural sense of confidence to your life.

5 CONFIDENCE BUILDING QUESTIONS
TO TURN ANXIETY INTO ACTION

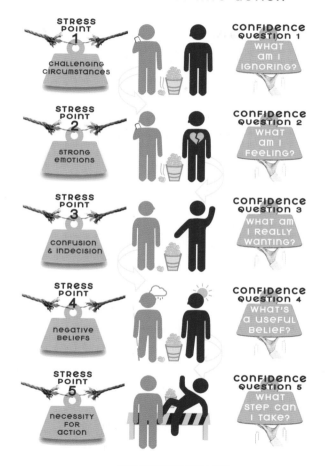

STRESS POINT 1
CHALLENGING CIRCUMSTANCES

CONFIDENCE QUESTION 1
WHAT AM I IGNORING?

STRESS POINT 2
STRONG EMOTIONS

CONFIDENCE QUESTION 2
WHAT AM I FEELING?

STRESS POINT 3
CONFUSION & INDECISION

CONFIDENCE QUESTION 3
WHAT AM I REALLY WANTING?

STRESS POINT 4
NEGATIVE BELIEFS

CONFIDENCE QUESTION 4
WHAT'S A USEFUL BELIEF?

STRESS POINT 5
NECESSITY FOR ACTION

CONFIDENCE QUESTION 5
WHAT STEP CAN I TAKE?

PART THREE

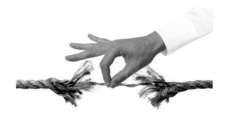

HOW TO TURN LIFE'S CHALLENGES TO YOUR ADVANTAGE

STRESS REDUCTION VS. STRESS PRODUCTION

In Part Two we discussed how to respond more usefully in the moment that stress arises. Here in Part Three we're going to look at a subtler layer of opportunity for building our confidence. These opportunities arise in the midst of our ordinary day-to-day challenges—challenges that we wouldn't even necessarily label as stressful because we've unconsciously found ways to steer around them in our daily lives. Here we will discuss what it looks like to steer *toward* those challenges and use the fuel they generate for confidence building.

Real confidence is built by using the presence of stress productively, turning it to our advantage rather than eliminating it. It's about stress *production* instead of stress *reduction*. It's about learning to surf on stress, like a wave we ride, rather than drowning in it to the detriment of our health and wellbeing.

We're going to discuss how we can benefit from the sensations of stress, rather than fear them and run away from them. A friend of mine, Stuart Goodnick, coined the wonderful phrase "follow your dread" to describe a practice he encourages as part of a mindfulness group he coleads for the Tayu Meditation Center in California. What does "follow your dread" mean, and why would anyone want to do it? In Stuart's words, following your dread refers to "getting in the grit of who we are and taking responsibility for the unconscious and mechanical manifestations that arise when we don't bring a responsible attention to the operation of our lives." In a nutshell—it's an invitation to stop ignoring the stuff that deserves our attention!

Trying to change other people, situations, and circumstances demonstrates our belief that stress is "out there," which makes it virtually impossible to take responsibility for the unconscious reactivity inside of us that undermines our faith in ourselves. As Goodnick's Tayu teaching partner, Rob Schmidt, pointed out in our recent interview, "We often feel that the deck is stacked against us in life, yet we fail to see that we ourselves have done the stacking."

I'm a member of an online listing service that matches speakers and entertainers with clients who are looking for performers. The following recent posting actually showed up as a request for services:

Looking for a magic act to perform for my wife. This magic act will serve as an apology from myself to her. Anywhere from 30 min. to 1 hour. Thanks.

We might imagine that this husband will be the one completely mystified when the magician fails to repair his relationship with his wife. Perhaps he rightly senses that he needs some real magic, something out of the ordinary to reconnect with his beloved. Such magic, however, is much more likely to arise from an act of authentic and direct communication than from some surrogate sleight of hand. One intriguing reference to the etymology of the word "abracadabra" identifies the Aramaic phrase *avra kadavra* as the origin of the word. *Avra kadavra* roughly translates as "it will be created in my words." Our words have enormous power, yet we fear using them for good. For this husband, magic could have been created from a few honest words, delivered vulnerably. Instead, he opts to send in an illusionist to handle the situation. We might say that magic occurs when we connect to truth, and illusion is what we get when we avoid the truth.

Stress avoidance as a relationship strategy usually culminates in looking for a new girlfriend or boyfriend, figuring we'll finally reduce our relationship stress when we find the "right" partner. As most of us well know, strong partnerships involve doubling down on honest communication when relatedness hits the rocks. This allows us to turn a rough patch into more trust and intimacy, rather than the reverse.

"Facing our dread" is often the shortest distance between big challenges and satisfying outcomes. Our mind, however, somehow convinces us of the impassibility of that direct route.

To consider making a sincere apology, for instance, might look to some of us like walking into a category-five hurricane. So we try to reduce our stress by actively ignoring things and situations that cause us discomfort, as we've previously discussed. We turn away from glaring truths and then express our dismay with the way things turn out. We are both our own magician and audience, performing masterful unconscious manipulations and then being amazed by what happens.

- We come late every day to work and then demand an explanation for why we are being fired.

- We constantly judge our partners and are surprised and hurt when they withdraw.

- We put no money in the meter and then curse the city when a ticket is waiting for us on the windshield.

- We babysit our children with screen time and then punish them when they're not responsive to us.

Intentional stress production is an entirely different way to live. It first involves complete acknowledgment of our outer and inner condition. We see our challenges as they are and see our own reactivity to those challenges as well. Then we use the energy of the stress to jump into life rather than avoid it. We learn to assert confidence even in the moments when our old intrusive feelings call for us to disengage.

An inspiring speaker named Troy Chambers, who recently presented after me on a conference platform, caught my attention from the moment he stepped on stage and lifted his trouser legs to show his comically bare ankles beneath his suit. He confessed to the nervousness that had left him a bit scattered in the departing moments of his trip, and thus without socks to wear. He then unhesitatingly launched into his presentation. The result was an instant connection with the audience, where a potential source of stress was embraced and served beautifully as a demonstration of connection and humanness.

Speaking with Chambers after his talk, I listened to him confide that he had gone to the front desk of the hotel, desperate for help in locating a pair of socks, and when they finally arrived moments prior to his introduction, he turned them down. He chose to be authentically present with his audience rather than scramble to cover the tracks of his true experience. It was a strong decision that illustrates the distinction between attempting to avoid stress and using it to delightful advantage. In this case, Troy Chambers's confidence in himself to be real with his audience translated into his audience having confidence in him.

A 2013 news story reported how a Yorkshire vicar facing mounting church repairs and a congregation that he had already tapped out for donations decided to give away ten-pound notes to all attending members of his church one day. In the face of being ultimately responsible for the church's maintenance, he loaded up the collection plates with the notes, totaling 550 English pounds, and told his parishioners they were free to do whatever they wanted with the cash. Just in case anyone was looking for ideas, he also suggested that the funds could be used as seed money for fundraising efforts. Ten thousand pounds, roughly a 2,000 percent gain on his creative investment, made its way back into the church coffers in the form of new contributions. Not a bad return for the simple act of demonstrating confidence in others!

Inner confidence arises from having faith in the workability of things as they are, trusting that the presence of a challenge is as likely to trigger an outbreak of our human ingenuity as it is an inescapable calamity.

Eleanor Roosevelt was the longest-serving First Lady in U.S. history, and perhaps one of the most productive. Every quote site on the Internet is brimming with her admonitions to face things as they are and get to work. One of her quotes I appreciate most is, "You gain strength, courage and confidence by every experience in which you really stop to look fear in the face. You must do the thing you think you cannot do."

Auguste Renoir, the famous impressionist painter whose works were already well known at the turn of the 20th century, painted for another twenty years after contracting severe rheumatoid arthritis. Despite the stress of ill health, Renoir remained a prolific and productive artist who simply summarized the secret of his success like this: "One must from time to time attempt things that are beyond one's capacity."

MANAGING AROUSAL

I met Katie at a recent training I led for the health services division of a California government agency. She told me a delightful story of a lifelong friend who "kidnapped" her on her thirty-second birthday. The vision that inspired the playful abduction was to steal Katie away from her "adult" life, fly her to another state (Florida), and invite her into activities meant to reinspire the youthful freedom that she and her friend had shared growing up. Included on the agenda were jumping in puddles, getting a massage (a first for Katie), raiding the backyards of strangers for fresh Florida fruit, butting into lineups, begging for change, and performing random acts of kindness for pedestrians.

The happiest and most fulfilled individuals among us share a secret demonstrated by Katie's childhood friend. To build confidence, we must challenge the habits we've acquired over time that we now mistake for our true limits. Katie's friend had an instinctive appreciation for intentional stressing. In the same vein, we're going to look at how "stressing smart" actually necessitates that we follow our dread, and how we can benefit from not just embracing, but even moving toward, the things we stress about.

Anyone who has the capacity to follow their dread is a kind of modern-day hero, many of whom are invisible leaders who parent patiently in the wee hours of the night, serve marginalized and forgotten members of the human race, or simply stretch themselves to respond with ordinary kindness, generosity, and compassion in the midst of a stressful world.

Following our dread may just look like continuing forward when we feel unprepared or unqualified or when our sense of identity is being challenged. Or it can show up as giving care and attention to someone we'd rather avoid. We can also dread wonderful things, like when a big break that we've always dreamed of suddenly shows up and we're then on the hook to walk our talk by making a significant stretch—physically, mentally, or emotionally.

Whether we perceive our stresses as being positive or negative, what happens to our stress levels when challenges are upon us? In the language of the early research of Yerkes-Dodson and the famous Yerkes–Dodson Law, we become aroused.[1]

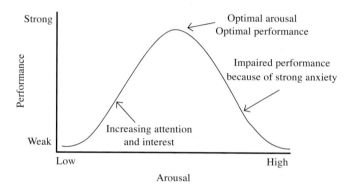

The research of Yerkes-Dodson confirms what we already know. When we care about something, we experience increased attention and interest. That leads to being more present, more engaged, and more effective in relation to the thing our attention is on. That is, until we "care" too much and our optimal responsiveness becomes eroded by excessive arousal, which we call *anxiety*.

THE THREE FUNDAMENTALS OF CONFIDENCE BUILDING

1. We need to get to know ourselves well enough through self observation, over time, to see where we usually "lose it" and our attention and interest turn into anxiety.

2. We must manage our environment and lifestyle to avoid exposing ourselves too much to our stress triggers so we can restore our opportunity for clear thinking.

3. We then need to practice moving toward the anxiety trigger in *small intentional ways* so we can start to be more conscious of this arousal and learn to act with confidence in the face of it, rather than becoming disabled by it.

Becoming aware of the anxious feelings that float in the background of our attention is vital work for anyone who wishes to experience the joy and fulfillment of true confidence in their life.

Everything we want for ourselves in the domains of money, health, and relationship depend upon the ability to fully experience all of our feelings as they are without getting overwhelmed by them. Increasing our capacity for this type of mindfulness is not easy work. And in addition to becoming aware enough to catch our reactivity as it occurs, we have to *take action. We need to prove to ourselves through direct experience that these old anxious feelings are not an accurate measure of our real limits.*

For instance, I often procrastinate when I need to be writing. Knowing in my mind that anxious feelings are the cause of my procrastination in writing makes zero difference; however, when I apply myself in action—writing a little bit each day and sharing it with others—my sense of feeling capable and powerful in my world is instantly and dramatically improved. In fact, years of engaging practice by taking action in the face of my anxiety is the only reason you're now reading this book. I took a previous run at this manuscript and shared my 40,000-word pride and joy with a small focus group. The result was a resounding "meh" and a shrug of collective shoulders. Cue the parade of anxious feelings. The only thing that kept me going was my practice of challenging my own personal precedent for collapsing in shame. And even at that, it took me nine months to get back on the horse and engage a complete overhaul of this book. But I did it and am personally very pleased with the result.

For every good book that reaches an audience, its history of edits contains enough poor writing to produce several bad ones. Consider that good books are produced by determined good authors, who are good because they care deeply about their work. Imagine the stress involved with having to write enough bad material to produce several terrible books in order to find your way to a useful one. That's *following one's dread* in a nutshell.

Is it hard work to overcome our old stress patterns and live more confidently? Yes! Does the hard work pale in comparison to how it feels to contribute our best to the world, to act in resonance with our most heartfelt wishes and grow more confident in our abilities day after day? Yes, again!

Now, perhaps you've tried other approaches in overcoming old limits, and lately you've given up because none of them have worked. There are two primary ways we fail to make progress in shedding old, self-doubting habits.

1. We invest in an awareness program that leaves us feeling calm, happy, and blissful when we're on the meditation cushion, enjoying our massage, speaking with our therapist, or getting high at the workshop, but we don't *practice the right action in our lives where it matters*, consistently over time, to anchor new behavior.

2. We introduce lots of new behavior in our lives over the top of our negative feelings without

fully *experiencing* those feelings. We run from self-awareness by chasing goal after goal, confusing achievement with growth as we avoid the emotional triggers that come back to haunt us, once again, if we ever slow down.

It's important that we understand the dynamics at play in scenario two. Many people fail to make a distinction between confidence and conquest. It's not unusual for a person to turn to conquest in an attempt to feel confident, when in fact they are simply covering up feelings of anxiety with an aggressive string of achievements. Unconsciously, this is an attempt to avoid what Dr. Geoffrey Carr calls *intrusive feelings*.

THE THREE INTRUSIVE FEELINGS

Dr. Geoffrey Carr is a clinical psychologist and author of the book *Making Happiness*.[2] I recently interviewed him regarding what he has termed "intrusive feelings." According to Dr. Carr, intrusive feelings are complex, but basically there are three types.

Type One is the feeling that something bad *is going* to happen. This is the feeling of fear. Fear comes in many flavors, such as anxiety, nervousness, worry, apprehension, panic, dread, and terror.

Type Two is the feeling that something bad *has happened*. This is the feeling of pain. We say we feel hurt, loss, sadness, longing, heartbreak, devastation, despair, or grief.

Type Three is the feeling that *we ourselves are somehow bad*. This is the feeling of shame. Shame includes feeling embarrassed, humiliated, guilty, inadequate, useless, repulsive, dirty, or flawed.

You probably know personally someone who has a talent, a skill, or something to offer that they delay taking action on and find excuses for not engaging. They have a book they're writing, an album they're producing, a small business they're starting, a stand-up routine they're working on, an important letter they haven't sent, a crucial project with a deadline, a résumé they plan on submitting, an art project they're creating—yet they're constantly finding reasons to run away from completing what they most want to accomplish.

I'm one of those people. Perhaps you are, too. What's really going on is that we're at the effect of intrusive feelings, a hidden stress that we're not educated to even see, much less manage. In my own case, I love to communicate. I'm also a performer, and writing is a type of performance for me. I care about how people respond to my performances and writing, which makes me prone to intrusive, fearful feelings about how my work will be received. The prospect of having my writing received unfavorably unconsciously prevents me from putting it out there. So I stall and come up with excuses, like having to check my email, even though the contribution I'm longing to offer to the world—and that would most fulfill me to provide—depends on sharing it! *These old intrusive feelings will shake our confidence every time unless we understand their nature, where they come from (the past), and have a plan for remaining committed and focused when they arise in our current adult lives.*

Dr. Carr also calls these intrusive feelings "stop" feelings, for an obvious reason. They stop us from moving toward anything that triggers them, because fear, pain, and shame don't feel good! The problem is, these feelings are *in us*, and to try to get away from them we ignore them and deny that they exist. The bigger problem is that ignoring works—*temporarily.* What we're left with is the burden of an avoidance pattern that is briefly relieving but leaves us feeling unprepared and doubtful of our abilities when it comes to handling our challenges and the internal distress that accompanies them. Living with confidence requires that we practice putting intrusive feelings into perspective. *They're just fear, pain, and shame.* They're not

- evidence of certain death.

- proof that we're cowards.

- a sign that we're bound to fail.

- a warning from God.

Confidence starts with the ability to see things as they are, and that includes our own internal feeling states, without assuming that we are bad and wrong for having them. Confidence is actively built when we are able to take appropriate adult action in the face of intrusive feelings.

INTELLIGENT MISBEHAVIOR

Awareness combined with the willingness to take action outside of limiting patterns is the magic formula. I call it *intelligent misbehavior*—presence combined with courageous action. More specifically, it is the practice of paying attention to our intrusive feelings, observing the patterns or rules that we cling to in the face of them, and then gently challenging those patterns in small ways, consistently over time, until new behaviors are established that allow us to engage rather than withdraw or back down from fully living. The action of such *intelligent misbehavior* is courageous because in order to take it we have to break old personal rules. These internal rules are an injunction against engaging with circumstances, activities, environments, and people similar to those that were present when we experienced a previous wounding.

The overall effect of these rules as they accumulate throughout our lives—from early childhood up through adulthood—is, unfortunately, a loss of confidence. The presence of the rules shrinks the types and kinds of experiences, opportunities, and relationships that we give ourselves permission to pursue. An example of this for me is making sales calls. As a self-employed speaker, there's no getting around the need to prospect leads and reach out to potential customers. My hate/love relationship with that task involves the fear of being rejected on one hand and the joy of getting paid to do what I love on the other. I can be perfectly aware of my fear, yet it's only picking up the phone and making contact that disrupts the grip of disabling stress and turns it into the joy of connecting with customers. In short, it's *awareness combined with action* that allows me to turn my stress around.

Imagine, for instance, that you are given this task of posing as a server for a banquet attended by 500 business professionals. In addition, your job is to purposefully annoy and irritate the dinner guests without letting on that it's all an act. You'd probably feel a little stressed in the face of the task, just as I do *every time* I have to put on a uniform and wade out into the crowd. This is an important point: The nervous feeling that I get when risking human contact *never fully goes away*— and yet I never hesitate to move into action in my job because I've proven to myself that my anxious feelings are not about *now*. My anxiety is the imprint of an old stress precedent that wants to limit my current life participation in the name of keeping me safe. If I were fixated on that feeling, I'd never be able to deliver my unique act. I'd be too scared to even try it.

On the other hand, if I tried to completely ignore the anxiety, it would find its footing with me unconsciously and I'd wind up finding excuses, good reasons, and justifications for not engaging that would sound rational, yet the underlying truth is that I'm just scared. The sweet spot is, I'm scared, but I'm going to challenge my fear with a little action, and see if my fear is valid. This method is how we liberate ourselves from a backlog of stress precedents that convinces us to "tap out" when we come up against any kind of stress. It's how we can transcend the habit of playing it safe, withdrawing, holding out, and avoiding risk in our lives. It's also how we discover which fears are actually useful, which cautions and concerns *are* about the present moment, and maturely protect our physical and emotional well-being without unnecessarily cutting ourselves off from life. As Helen Keller once said, "Life is either a bold adventure, or nothing at all."

Little by little and step by step, not expecting to transcend all of our rules at once, we can slowly and surely approach that bold adventure ourselves. In fact, there is no power on earth that can stop us once we learn the practice of *intelligent misbehavior*. For a more detailed look at some cultural rules that we all tend to follow, to our detriment, you may want to refer to my previous book on the subject, *7 Rules You Were Born to Break*.

SMALL ACTIONS, BIG RESULTS

Dr. Sian Beilock is an associate professor in the department of psychology at the University of Chicago. She is an expert on performance and brain science and author of the recent book *Choke: What the Secrets of the Brain Reveal About Getting It Right When You Have To*. Dr. Beilock's book is an important contribution to our world at a time when the pressures of modern-day life have never been greater. Drawing upon a prodigious body of recent research, she details how students, athletes, and business professionals can improve their performance when the pressure is on. In all instances, the solution to being at our best in the throes of stress involves one thing: practice.

The good news is that small amounts of practice can make more of a difference than we might suspect. Dr. Beilock cites the work of Raôul Oudejans, who is with the MOVE Research Institute at Vrije University in Amsterdam and whose recent focus has been supporting law enforcement officials to function effectively in high-pressure situations. Dr. Beilock summarizes Oudejans's finding for us.

> [E]ven practicing under mild levels of stress can prevent people from falling victim to the dreaded choke when high levels of stress come around.
>
> When people practice in a casual environment with nothing on the line and are then put under pressure to perform well…they often choke under the pressure. But if people practice…with some mild stressors to begin with…their performance doesn't suffer when the big stressors come around.[3]

I was in a second-hand bookshop recently and ran across a self-help paperback with the message "*This book changed my life!*" written across the cover by the previous owner. No book, however, ever changes our lives. We could argue that the best books change our *minds*, yet in order for the ideas they present to change our *lives,* we have to act. Not only that, we have to act with confidence in a moment that counts. The moments that count are those moments when we will be tempted to do the old thing, yet find the wherewithal to engage a new choice.

We're not generally triggered into flight, fight, or freeze mode when we're engrossed in a book or listening to a motivational speaker. As we all know, once we're faced with our daily challenges again it's a lot harder to access the potential we glimpsed while we were listening to the passionate speaker or engrossed in our inspiring book. We all want to feel that potential. The fact is, we don't tend to feel it when we're actually being confronted by our stress triggers in the midst of our challenging lives. This makes us want to get back into the audience again—read another book or attend another seminar. After all, that's where we felt so good! The problem is, we can't *practice* real life from the audience. We can only practice usefully when we have "something on the line," as Raôul Oudejans puts it. To fully realize what a good author or speaker helps us to glimpse, we have to practice in the presence of stress. Books don't change our lives; *we do* when we take courageous action in the presence of intrusive feelings.

On my way to catch a flight one morning, my cab driver was driving dangerously, aggressively riding the bumpers of the cars in front of us at high speed in heavy traffic. It was very stressful for me to find the courage to tell him what I thought of his driving and ask him to slow down. It took most of the ride for me to speak up. What was on the line in that moment for me was the feeling that something bad would happen if I told the taxi driver that I didn't approve of his driving. I wanted the taxi driver to like me, and I tend to avoid any kind of interaction that might cast me in a negative light.

You might find that silly and perhaps would have had no problem communicating your concerns and boundaries. Likely, there are other situations that would stress you out and wouldn't bother another person at all. Each of us is different, and each of us has different work to do in relation to the life areas where we lose our confidence.

Stress tends to show up where we have a strong desire for things to go well. Our need to have things be a certain way is backed by a strong belief that our happiness, safety, and success depend upon the world cooperating with our plan. The point here is that we must be willing to engage with people and circumstances when they *don't* conform to our rulebook, when they're *not* under our total control. We have to move toward things that we'd typically like to avoid, but we only have to do it in small ways. Research shows us that practicing in small ways can lead to big results. As Dr. Beilock tells us in her book, "Practice can actually change the wiring of the brain to support exceptional performance.[4] Just as lifting weights helps to develop your bicep muscles, practice shapes your brain."[5]

If we're honestly observing ourselves, we'll get to know where our sore spots are and where intrusive feelings arise. Once we've done that, we can engage in a kind of habit engineering where we redesign our behavior to gently meet—rather than avoid—the triggers that produce our stress. Yet, it all starts with just paying more careful attention to our lives.

YOUR ATTENTION IS BETTER THAN A GP'S DEGREE

We've already discussed in Part Two how essential the quality of presence is to our capacity for confidence. If we want to be able to handle the ordinary moments of our lives successfully and the stressful moments usefully, we have *to be there*! When we are following a reactive chain of thoughts, we're leading ourselves away from the present moment, setting ourselves up to fail at handling it well, and then having our sense of self-confidence become diminished based on the evidence of those failures.

Several years ago I badly damaged my shoulder, but I didn't know how. It was completely messed up. I experienced severe pain with any movement of my right arm and had extremely limited mobility. I couldn't raise my elbow at all, yet it was a mystery to me how and why this had occurred. I went to my doctor, who examined me and told me he'd seen this before. "Frozen shoulder," he called it. He said I was facing at least six months of physical therapy to get the use of it back. He told me to take Advil to help keep the inflammation down until I could see the physiotherapist he was scribbling out a referral for.

It's tempting for us all to invest more confidence in some sort of expert, degreed professional, or authority figure than we reserve for ourselves and our own ability to pay attention and take charge of our own health or other aspects of our lives. In this circumstance, I was torn between bowing to authority and heeding what my gut was saying. I heard the diagnosis that came from my doctor, but it didn't make sense to me. Why had I suddenly developed this shoulder problem? I'm quite active, so yes, my arms are in use a lot, but there was no memorable incident to explain what I was experiencing.

Days passed while I slowly accepted that this had somehow happened and that I should get help. I made the appointment with the physiotherapist, who added me to a long list of patients who were scheduled several weeks out. Still, I couldn't get this puzzle out of my mind. Something wasn't right, and I was determined to figure out what it was, so I started closely watching my movements and actions. I'm a writer and communicator and I do a lot of work in my home office, particularly on the computer. I had been through a work period where jobs were thin and money was tight. I was stressed. Then one day I noticed that I had developed a habit of slumping forward onto my desk, propping myself up in a mood of despondency. It would have looked something like this (without the pretty hair).

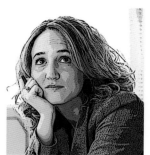

Now, this was a nondramatic, ordinary action that I probably engaged hundreds of times a day without noticeable impact. Yet, the cumulative effect of repeatedly bearing the weight of my heavy feelings eventually created a big problem for my shoulder joint! The moment I realized what I had been doing, the light bulb went off and I felt a rush of euphoria. I knew immediately this was the problem. I remained vigilant in watching my posture and stopped myself every time I was about to lean on my arm. In a week, my shoulder was completely freed up, and I've been fine ever since!

This incident showed me two things.

1. How small, low-grade habits, repeated over time, can hurt us or heal us.

2. If we're suffering, it behooves us to invest our confidence first in our own attention and look at the small stuff before we start seeing doctors, spending money, taking drugs, having surgery,

visiting therapists, going on wild diets, and looking for other external "fixes."

It's up to us to experiment with natural, close to home, basic observations and changes as a first course of action—testing for ourselves what might be contributing to our challenge.

What if many of our stumbling blocks and stresses were actually arising from the repetition of small unconscious actions that are flying under our radar? What if learning to manage our own attention and applying it confidently to our problems could make a bigger difference in the quality of our lives than anything else we could do?

If this were so, then two things would be true.

1. Management of our own attention and our ability to self observe would be the most precious and important resource we could develop.

2. An "expert," doctor, or other professional would be less likely to be able to help us than we ourselves are, since no one else is with us in the context of long-term, attentive, and interested daily observation.

Our doctor can detect leukemia, but no doctor can detect the repeated micro-movements of attention that trigger us into patterns of tension and dis-ease that can affect not only our entire physical system, but our emotions, relationships, and sense of potential. As best-selling author Dr. Gabor Maté reminds us, "In healing, every bit of information, every piece of the truth may be crucial."[6]

Now, I'm *not* saying that you should never see doctors or specialists, but I am saying, don't expect that they have all the answers! Our life challenges—and the creative means by which we can rewire ourselves to have those challenges serve us rather than disable us—must have our own personal, fully committed attention. We have to become confident in our own observational capacity and be willing to apply it. With such observation we'll have the opportunity to begin designing new habit routines for ourselves that make huge differences in our lives. These new routines will fall into two categories.

1. Small things we stop doing that have been undermining us—like abdicating important decisions to those we deem to be authority figures instead of staying present to our own challenges.

2. Small things we start doing: speaking up when we disagree with a decision or a point of view, for example.

In both cases, the goal is to start trusting ourselves a little more by committing to small actions of confidence on a regular basis.

GROWTH WAITS BEHIND THE DOOR OF DISTURBANCE

By nature, we humans do not move toward things that produce discomfort or anxiety in us, or that pose some degree of challenge to our habits and perceptions. "And...?" you may be wondering. "What's wrong with that?"

The problem is that our growth and potential are often hidden behind that door of disturbance. It's disturbing to stop overeating, let our kids make their own mistakes, turn off the television and take a real-life risk, or get out of bed early and get to the gym. Yet, we have to be willing to open the door to such challenges, be with those stressful elements, and brave them to get the benefit of living better lives and brighter futures. The same signals that light up warning signs that tell us to "stay away" from certain circumstances and people can also be road markers of opportunity, contribution, and profound connection.

I was recently playing in the park with my son when a woman pulled up next to the playground in her car to take a phone call. As we continued playing, the call went on and on. All the while, her car was idling right there on the curbside. I'm not one to mind other people's business. (Not out loud anyway.) Any potential for confrontation sends me in the other direction. Yet, it was hard to ignore the greenhouse emissions from her aging vehicle as it pumped exhaust into the atmosphere. I really wanted to ask her to turn off her car, yet also feared what her reaction might be.

After much internal wrestling, I eventually approached the passenger side of the car, and when she looked over, I mimed the act of turning off the ignition. She looked confused at first, and then, when my communication registered, she immediately shut down the engine, smiled a big smile and, looking apologetic, silently mouthed the words "Thank you" as she continued with her call. Phew!

If each of us were to add up the number of human conversations we've avoided, we'd have quite a list. And we'll never know how many lives, careers, opportunities, or wounded feelings we could have saved if we'd taken those risks. It is undoubtedly true that some challenging conversations actually *are* best to avoid. Yet, if we fearfully avoid *all* of them, we can never develop the intelligence that allows us to discriminate between reasonable risks of engagement and conversations that could be more usefully pursued at another time.

Some people credit Hans Selye as being the first scientist to demonstrate the existence of biological stress.[7] The Hungarian-Canadian endocrinologist made a distinction back in 1975 between stress and distress when he coined the term "eustress"—consisting of the Greek prefix *eu-*, meaning "good," and *stress*—literally meaning "good stress." Eustress introduced the concept of beneficial stress and the possibility that an individual might not only be able to accommodate stress, but to actually increase his or her confidence and capacity as a result of engaging it.

Stress signals can be growth signals or stop signs, depending on who we are and what we believe about our ability to handle challenges. The research of psychologist Carol Dweck studied the growth disparities between "growth mindset" individuals and "fixed mindset" individuals—the growth mindset group being those who believe they can learn from challenges and mistakes rather than believing their abilities are fixed.[8] As you'd imagine, the research demonstrated that people with a confident mindset outgrow those who have a fixed perspective of their abilities. Similarly, the predominant mindset regarding stress is that it's debilitating. We unconsciously defend ourselves against challenges without realizing how it strands us on an island of unrealized potential.

Justin Menkes, author of the Harvard Business Review book *Better Under Pressure*, wrote,

> *Human beings are not naturally wired to engage in complex problem solving when they are under pressure, but it can be learned. [Aspiring leaders] need to gain experience in stressful situations where they get an elevated—but not overwhelming—sense of adrenaline and are set up for success. Confidence under pressure can be built like a railroad track in the brain through exposure to repeated experiences over time.*[9]

In the same vein, this book, *Confident Under Pressure*, is an invitation to train ourselves to start stressing smarter, and you don't need to be an aspiring leader to reap the benefits. Just wanting to lead our own lives with more inner authority and confidence is a good enough reason to start practicing *intelligent misbehavior*, wisely breaking those personal rules that do nothing but hold us back.

Perhaps you remember a time when you've cancelled an interview for a new job, backed away from expressing a concern or a passion, stayed in bed for days after a loss, or fumed for weeks over a single comment made in passing. Perhaps you've even dodged somebody you know by ducking into a grocery store aisle and pretending to be completely absorbed in a search for pickles. (No? Okay, I guess that's just me.) In any case, there's a way out of such entertaining, but ultimately life-limiting, behavior. You too can navigate the presence of ordinary stress in a smarter and more useful way.

Driving past a local park near my home one day, I ran into a traffic lineup on a picturesque back street, a route that I intentionally took to avoid the routine congestion of the city and to enjoy the scenery. I was irritated by the slowdown, even though "slowing down" was my original motivation. At a standstill, working with my reaction to the gridlock, I noticed a woman run up to the driver-side window of the vehicle two cars ahead of me, lean forward to say something, and then quickly withdraw to approach the driver directly in front of me. She repeated the process, and I was going to be next. I had no idea what she might say to me.

As she ran to my open window she simply asked one question with utter urgency: "Do you have any allergy medication?!"

I was confused, but said no, and she immediately ran to the car behind me. I watched in my rearview mirror as she worked her way down the line—focused, clear, active in her mission to find an EpiPen, presumably.

A minute or two later, as traffic began to move, I looked over to my right at the edge of the park, where a young man was lying on the ground, evidently the victim of an allergic reaction. His bike had fallen next to him. He had apparently been traveling through the park alone at the onset of his attack. But he wasn't alone now. He was surrounded by nine other people who were standing around staring at him, immobilized by dread, doing nothing!

The difference between the person who was sprinting down the street from car to car, unapologetically bringing traffic to a standstill, and those who stood doing nothing is just one thing: training. And you can bet that if it wasn't formal first-responder training this woman had, it was some form of modeling in her life that taught her how to respond confidently in a challenging circumstance rather than freeze. She had either seen or personally practiced confidence under pressure. She had a stress precedent in place that said, "I've seen this handled before," or "I've survived it before," or "There's something I can do." And such enabling precedents come from practice: participating in and advancing from small to larger challenges in life while learning to stay present, access real feeling, identify a purpose, imagine a possibility, and get in motion.

The contrast between the inaction of the bystanders, and even my own petty irritation with the traffic jam, and the full-fledged service of this bright and confident woman brought me to tears. It was a vivid demonstration of the difference between living and the mood of fearful hesitation that enshrouds most of us in its fog from day to day. It's the repeated application of low-level *intelligent misbehavior* that prepares us for such service where it matters.

Once, between speaking appearances, I had to catch a train between two New England cities. It was rush hour and the train was full.

I sat down next to a young gentleman who looked like he wanted to be left alone. I just wanted to be left alone too, but the seats were all full, so I took 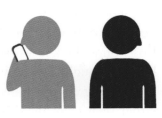 the spot next to him. Sitting there, I realized that this small circumstance of having to sit close to another person was stressful for me.

I had two choices: ignore him and say nothing for the forty-minute trip, or strike up a conversation. Of course, there's no guarantee that he would want to talk, and the idea of trying to start a conversation and having the other person reject the overture is stressful. But just sitting four inches from another human being and trying to ignore them is stressful, too. So I decided to take the risk and say hello. As it turned out, we had a lively and interesting conversation about stress!

He was traveling for work as well, on his way to sort out a mess with a construction project in another city. I talked about my book project, and he wanted to 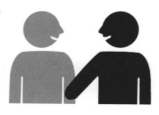 know more. Consequently, the forty-minute ride felt like two minutes. Had I just gritted my teeth and tried to ignore this person, it would have felt like two hours.

This is where real life happens. As inspiring as the big stories of fast-acting heroes are, it's the small moments of our lives where we can make the biggest difference and experience the most personal fulfillment. When self-defeating feelings arise, tempting us to make the decision to shrink away from our lives, and we instead make the choice to challenge them with an action of confidence, we thrive.

Again, awareness alone is often not enough to loosen the grip of our old patterns. We need to *practice behaving* in ways that demonstrate the freedom we actually have to participate and act in our lives. The key is not to expect too much, but just make the effort to lean in a small way against the defensive habit of backing away from action and participation. This is so important that I need to say it one more time.

Awareness, combined with the willingness to take action outside of limiting patterns, is the winning formula for building confidence.

GAMES FOR CONFIDENCE

In her latest book, *Why Motivating People Doesn't Work and What Does*, author and researcher Susan Fowler describes the three psychological needs of a human being and how—when these needs are met—an individual enjoys a perpetual, free-flowing source of motivation for living their best life. The third psychological need she addresses is *competence*. In Fowler's words, "Competence is our need to feel effective at meeting everyday challenges and opportunities. It is demonstrating skill over time. It is feeling a sense of growth and flourishing."[10]

Developing competence in relation to stress and becoming effective at meeting everyday challenges is our entire focus in this book. Such competence is the key to maintaining confidence under pressure.

So, how do we attain competence? The same way our children learn to walk. By stumbling forward with *incompetence*, learning from our direct experience and mastering one challenge at a time. If we throw ourselves into intensely challenging circumstances, where the stakes are high and our competence is low, we'll have to peel ourselves off the floor of the Yerkes-Dodson curve due to our resulting impaired performance and high anxiety.

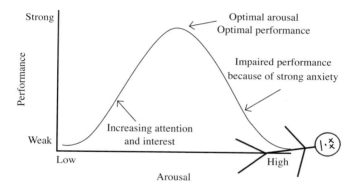

What we're looking for is a balance of arousal that activates our learning spirit without overstimulating our limbic alarms. If we manage this kind of training properly, we can actually lift the threshold of our arousal capacity and enjoy ever-increasing freedom to engage more demanding and fulfilling challenges in life.

I've invented something called *Games for Confidence* for myself to engage such training on a regular basis. *Games for Confidence* are *intentional investments in small disturbances that prepare us for an ever-increasing degree of competence.*

This entire book is literally worth nothing to us if we don't actually engage in small actions of *intelligent misbehavior*. We cannot think our way out of the limiting patterns of our stress precedents. In further instruction from Stuart Goodnick, he clarifies that message: "Following your dread is not a cognitive process. In fact, it is a process that is designed to *confound* the cognitive process."

The *idea* of trickling water over stone didn't create the Grand Canyon over millions of years. The *act* of it did. It is repeated, consistent, limit-expanding action that counts for growth, and it only takes minor adjustments in our behavior to make a big difference over time. Small actions taken with new confidence are the key. They don't take a lot of time, they don't require a great amount of motivation, they don't trigger the defenses of the people around us who have gotten used to our usual habits, and they can be sustained *over time*. Stephen Guise, author of the popular book *Mini Habits,* clarifies this point beautifully.

> *Repetition has always been the one and only way for humans to intentionally [mold] the subconscious to their liking.* Mini Habits *took this basic*

> *truth and drew the logical conclusion that consis-*
> *tency mattered more than anything else, including*
> *goal size. If consistency matters most, and it does*
> *for habit-related pursuits, smaller goals are always*
> *superior because they are easier to do consistently.*[11]

So, small actions taken with new confidence on a regular basis . . . It all sounds clear and simple; however, this is not an easy task. Showing up in a *responsive* manner where we used to *react* is one of the most demanding challenges we can engage. If we expect to make that shift all at once, we're going to wind up disappointed. Our habits are dogged. It would be naïve to imagine that we can unravel the force of our defense mechanisms without a significant measure of persistent, self-compassionate effort. It doesn't happen all at once. We need to fight habit fire with habit ice. Habit ice is the patient, glacial-moving force of our unwavering intention and repeated small action.

Marshall Goldsmith is the author of the *New York Times* bestseller *What Got You Here Won't Get You There.* In his book, Goldsmith describes how numerous unexamined micro-habits that we're culturally prone to act out can create a primary barrier to professional success, especially for aspiring executives. Our biological programming, however, hasn't read Goldsmith's book.

We are evolutionarily designed for fierce loyalty to our existing habit patterns, because they've kept us alive so far! The psychophysical organism must be subjected to a great deal of repetitive training to be taught new tricks.

I first encountered this truth in my early life as a young athlete passionately interested in sports, and then in my teen years when I entered the performing arts. Extensive training in gymnastics, years of learning circus skills, and a few years as a member of a ballet company all demonstrated the need and value of discipline with respect to learning new behavior. By the time I turned my attention to inner growth, I already understood that any improvements I could make would occur incrementally, and only through the application of repeated practice . . . especially if the changes I sought were backed by the emotional force of old stress precedents.

Strong stress precedents create the perception that our survival is at stake, and they arm our unconscious habit-commitments with formidable resolve. We all have our own battalion of inner-change police who are ready to squash any new-habit uprising at a moment's notice. Small, slow, gradual changes do not summon their need to thwart our forward progress.

An example of the power of unconscious habit-commitments showed up when I entered a training program to lead a personal growth weekend. I had personally received so much from the program after being a participant myself that I wanted to facilitate it for others. Throughout the training period the instructor and other participants pointed out that the moment real feelings showed up in the room I would find some way to make a joke out of the circumstance. When first confronted with this observation I was defensive and dismissive of the idea that there was a problem. To me, it seemed like a perfectly useful response, turning seriousness into laughter.

The true underpinnings of the pattern were less benign. I had grown up in a family where logic ruled and I had become a "funny guy," and later the "class clown," as a way to make sure that no one's feelings got the upper hand. Why? Because I had not developed my own competency to handle feelings; therefore, I lost my confidence when they arose. My own discomfort with feelings created the need to deflect all opportunities for vulnerability in the face of emotion. I also used this joking form of passive aggression to dominate and control the space, instead of cleanly expressing anger when I felt it.

After a while I started to see the aggression that was involved in derailing present work in the room with the distraction of "humor." Repeatedly, I would react with dismay when I'd make a joke and have it pointed out that I'd done it again. My blindness to the habit became its own joke, as I'd fall into the behavior repeatedly. Only after a few weeks of continuous sessions did I actually began to notice this process in action. I'd still be taken over by the old habit and make the joke, but eventually I could see it *as* it happened. A little later, I was able to catch myself just *before* I made the joke, and with some difficulty manage to refrain. Now, decades later, I mostly manage the impulse to use humor to dissipate the presence of my own or others' feelings. What remains is my ability to apply my sense of humor in appropriate and useful ways, confident that I can handle the presence of my own feelings or those of others.

In short, building confidence requires time, and a large measure of succeeding comes from managing the expectations we're holding for our own progress. If we tend to lose our confidence when we're having an argument with someone, for instance, we might start to track one small manifestation of these encounters— like the habit of interrupting the other person in our attempt to take control of the conversation. We could have a goal of not interrupting them *just once* during the next argument we have, even though we really want to jump in and say something. The next time we argue, we might try to refrain from interrupting twice. Then three times. If we're able to achieve that kind of shift, as small as it is, that's worthwhile progress.

To refrain from correcting others, or "proving" them wrong when we feel our very survival depends upon doing so, is a challenge. Holding our tongue just once is a small disturbance we invest in to move toward the greater rewards afforded by respectful relationship. We are disrupting our old stress precedent with this small mindful action.

What I've just described is a *Game for Confidence*. Over the years, I have trained myself in many different disciplines involving both inner and outer skill sets. In the process, I've learned how to engineer precisely defined practices I can follow that will get me to where I want to go. In *The Power of Habit*, Charles Duhigg refers to these as *keystone habits*: single individual actions that, when performed, positively impact a collection of associated behaviors.[12] Like how quitting smoking could lead to eating better and exercising more. Or watching less television could lead to a better night's sleep.

When we work with making a small change to a stress reaction, we lessen the grip that reaction has on us. Interrupting others, for example, is a manifestation of the stress reaction *Ignoring Reality*. When we simply refrain from interrupting, we take responsibility for our inner reactivity, for bearing it, and in the process prove to ourselves that we don't have to discount the truth of others to survive. Such an ability to be with things as they are gives us an enormous sense of confidence. Each time we challenge an old stress reaction by refraining from an action we believe we *must* take, or by taking a small action that we believe we *must not* take, we reduce the influence that our stress precedents have on us and start to free ourselves from old behavioral commandments. Again, self-confidence is the result.

After many years of observing my own mechanics, I started designing simple practices, keystone habits for stress, that I could exercise in the flow of an ordinary day to turn subtle forms of stress reactivity into increased responsiveness. As I began to watch for reactive subtleties in myself I was absolutely amazed at the number of hiding places we have for stress reactivity that is considered normal and acceptable by cultural standards. Many good examples show up in Marshall Goldsmith's book *What Got You Here Won't get You There*, which I referred to earlier.

Such hidden stress-harbors as

- starting a sentence with the words "no," "but," or "however."

- making excuses.

- withholding information.

These little habits are ways in which we try to control others in our environment rather than developing our confidence to relate to our lives and to others as they are.

THE ENEMY INSIDE

Here's a fascinating account of reactivity in the pro sports domain involving what is commonly referred to as "trash talk." In 1998, in a typical game of Monday night football that took place between the Kansas City Chiefs and the Denver Broncos, the Broncos led as the Chiefs initiated their final touchdown drive. But the effort went sharply south as the Chiefs were flagged five times for unsportsmanlike conduct. What happened?

Trash talk refers to the verbal sparring that takes place in virtually all competitive sports, where a player attempts, in the words of Hall of Fame inductee Warren Sapp, to "[take] somebody's mind away from the task at hand."[13] Of the five penalties thrown at the Chiefs in that football game, Hall of Fame pass rusher Derrick Thomas was single-handedly responsible for three of them.

As it turned out, Shannon Sharpe, a leading American football tight end for the opposing Broncos, was not just talented at catching touchdown passes. He also excelled at trash talk. And on this particular occasion, he preyed upon a hidden stress-weakness in Thomas by memorizing the phone number of Thomas's girlfriend and reciting it to him one digit at a time, play by play, inciting Thomas to retaliate rather than focus on the game. In post-game comments, Thomas confessed,

I allowed a situation to get out of hand. For that, I apologize to my teammates who were on the field with me. I jeopardized our ability to win a football game. I sincerely apologize and say to them my actions of last evening will never occur again.

And to his young fans Thomas added,

To the youth of America that look up to Derrick Thomas, I apologize to you because that is not sportsmanlike conduct and you should not conduct yourself that way on the field.[14]

A compelling apology and promise from a star athlete, who by all standards had trained himself to respond to all the physics of NFL stress like a champion. He was an impressive specimen of physical stamina, strength, and persistence. Underneath all that highly trained muscle, however, lurked an unaddressed stress-weakness called "emotions." As prepared as this athlete was for the visible stresses of his professional challenge, he wasn't fully prepared for the *internal stress* of his own emotional triggers and perceptions. This example is instructive as to how you and I get thrown off our game in daily life.

I've invented innumerable ways, for instance, to procrastinate on getting this book into print. Just the other day I turned my computer on, intending to head straight to my writing, and thought to myself, "I'm going to get to this writing in just a minute, but first…" and I checked my email. In a horror movie, that moment in which I opened my email would have been when the eerie, creepy backtrack started to play, just the way it does when a really dumb film character slowly reaches out with one hand to open the basement door in the old abandoned house once belonging to a dead serial killer. Everyone watching is thinking, "You idiot! *Do not* open that door! Can't you hear the music?!" Well, that was me as I navigated to my mail app and opened Pandora's inbox. Before long I was lost in unsatisfying busy work.

I'm not going to even bother to ask if you've done this: used "but first" as a way to procrastinate taking action on a useful or important task. The tendency is universally human. We all deflect ourselves from taking meaningful action at one time or another. If you haven't used email as a distraction before, you probably don't own a computer.

There are ways other than checking email that tempt us to shy away from our important focus. You may have done it by opening the refrigerator door—or a copy of the *National Enquirer*. The odd thing is that we even distract ourselves with things that will help us, that are good for us, and sometimes with things that we love.

Indeed, I actually love to write! Similarly, there are probably things you actually enjoy doing once you're in motion with them, yet you may have wondered, "Why do I put off and delay the activities that are healthy, satisfying, meaningful and useful to me?" The answer is that we fail to account for the internal stress of our emotional triggers and perceptions. And those triggers are accompanied by a particular kind of trash talk. The way Derrick Thomas lost his focus on the football is actually not much different from how you and I lose our focus in daily life.

You're probably good at what you do, whether it's parenting, administrating, managing and leading, selling, creating or producing the right results at your job, just like Derrick. In your own domain, you're a well-trained, high-functioning machine. Now imagine, for a moment, squaring off at the line of scrimmage in an

NFL game, with an opponent who was every bit your equal in size and strength. An opponent whose committed focus is to stop you from advancing toward your goal. In the world of football, the things that linebackers say to each other as they're nose to nose, waiting for the ball to snap into play, can make all the difference between a run to the Super Bowl and a nosedive to the bottom of the NFL standings. Now consider that, in your real life, the same thing is going on. You are, in fact, always nose to nose with an opposing part of yourself that doesn't want you to advance, at the same time as you believe that you are dedicated and committed to your goals. In short, you trash talk another part of yourself: "This will never work." "They're going to see right through you." "They're paying you more than you're worth." "You screwed this up last time and you'll probably mess it up again."

Of course, I've only dramatized an internal character that perhaps you recognize. Part of the problem we face on the field of life is that our inner opposition is a silent foe. Its disempowering taunts are whispered and repeated so often that we've just stopped consciously listening to them. Unconsciously, however, they keep coming as relentless waves of unchecked assault on our sense of confidence: "Who do you think you are?" "You're not good enough." "Now would be a good time to quit, before you make a fool of yourself."

Not only does this self-directed trash talk prevent us from performing at our best, it sometimes goads us into delivering our worst. Once again, we have to work with these disabling habits in a conscious manner. *Games for Confidence* consist of small, regular efforts we make to stand up to those old voices inside of us that want us to fold on the field. Like my practice of writing, even in the face of my own trash-talking inner critic.

I've created hundreds of specific practices over the years that get to the heart of many of the hidden cultural rules we suffer from. I've also tested them with focus groups of more than one thousand people. In Part Four, I'm going to share with you a few examples of the games that others found most useful.

PART FOUR

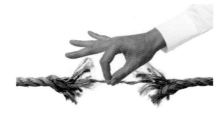

GAMES FOR CONFIDENCE

Developing Confidence of Presence
Game 1 – Games for Confidence
Information Fast for a Day

There are two ways to attend more actively to our present circumstance and receive all that it has to offer us: 1. Fill our perception with the subjects and objects that anchor our attention in the present moment, and 2. *Refrain* from placing our attention on the subjects and objects that lead us away from the present moment. This *Game for Confidence* uses the second method: guarding our attention from being eaten by distractions.

One such major distraction is *information*. Here's a way to work with the tendency to get carried away by information: Pick a day of your choice and, for its duration, ignore any information that is not directly relevant to your present and current activity. That means you'll probably be "fasting" from most all of your social media posts and 99 percent of mainstream news unless a tornado approaches your neighborhood and you need to access broadcast information about the nearest points of refuge.

You may also find yourself having to bypass even more local news, including information surrounding you on the job that is not directly necessary for you to know in the course of the day's work—like lingering over the copy machine so you can eavesdrop on the conversation your coworker is having with your supervisor. Instead, you'll move on to your present business. Nor will you stay on the phone with a friend or neighbor as they launch into some juicy gossip about their own or someone else's relationship issues. Fascinating articles, alluring headlines, the newspaper sitting on the doorstep, ads, commercials—give yourself a chance to be *here* and let them all be irrelevant to you for a day.

A large measure of our distraction comes from paying undue attention to facts and information we can do nothing about. This takes our attention away from the immediate needs of our environment and from attending to our current purpose in life. Minimizing information distraction provides us with a chance to remember where we are, what's really occurring around us, and what we want to be up to. The news about "current events" actually removes our attention from the real current events right where we are and in our own personal experience.

Beta Test Responses from Participants

Friday I spent the afternoon with my daughter and a girlfriend of mine. We went to lunch. Then later that evening I went to dinner with that girlfriend,

her husband and children. We had a nice time and I didn't watch the news or read the paper. I played Scrabble with her sons. It was a very nice, relaxing, and conversing day. It made me realize how taking in all that information from the world makes me stressed out and overwhelmed. Great exercise!
—CD

This was a huge challenge as every evening and morning the first thing that goes on is the news! I didn't listen to any news all weekend and it was so refreshing. I heard news from others talking about the weather back east, and my response was, "I didn't hear about that." It was nice to stay focused on what was around me. —VF

What a great day! No TV or talk radio was really cool. I didn't feel the stresses of the world. I was better able to connect with my family, as well. We are going to take regularly scheduled breaks from now on! —JD

DEVELOPING CONFIDENCE OF EMOTION
GAME 2 – GAMES FOR CONFIDENCE
ELIMINATE "I THINK"

As we come into closer contact with the reality of our feeling lives, it's beneficial to practice being accurate and honest about what we're experiencing. A simple way to cultivate our own self-awareness is to pay attention to the language we use when we're expressing ourselves; for instance, to not use "I think" when we really mean "I feel." "I think that's a bad idea" might then become "I feel afraid this is going to fail." "I think you're wrong" might become "I'm sad you see this differently." The next time you notice the phrase "I think" about to cross your lips, consider substituting the words "I feel…" followed by a communication that more accurately conveys the truth of your position, perspective, or experience.

Eliminating "I think" is a way of getting closer to our experience and communicating more transparently. We can always change our position if our thoughts do not find agreement; however, when we declare what we feel, and others don't feel the same way, we're exposed to the potential for intrusive feelings. While speaking our truth places us in a more vulnerable position, it also puts us in a position of greater clarity and personal strength. This can create an exhilarating shift of experience as we tap directly into what has been a previously unavailable energy source.

As always, what we choose to express to others deserves intelligence and discretion. It's not always necessary or useful to share our innermost feelings with everybody. There are times, however, when being self-revealing is useful and even inspiring to others. If we never experiment with this type of courageous expression we miss the opportunity to learn skillful means in this area, and it becomes easier for us to lose track of the power that comes from our feeling reality.

Beta Test Responses from Participants

I was able to practice this one on Saturday with my husband. I often start statements with "I think you should…" so I changed some of those statements to "I feel that this might be a better way to handle…" and since he is kind-hearted (tough exterior) I think he listened to me more than I'm used to. What can I say…this could become a new trend for me! —KM

This practice brought to light how much I discount what I feel. It was running through my head all day that it is okay to feel strongly about something.

I had one opportunity to switch "I feel" for "I think" and it made me feel good to be more authentic! I gave some advice to an applicant who was using our online recruitment software and he seemed to appreciate it. —TM

DEVELOPING CONFIDENCE OF VISION
GAME 3 – GAMES FOR CONFIDENCE
SKIP THE APPROVAL

This practice involves identifying an action, goal, or initiative that you're interested in pursuing, yet are acting as though you require approval from someone else before you proceed. Just identify one thing you are excited to engage that you don't actually need anyone's approval to move toward.

Unconsciously, we often use the idea of needing some kind of permission to buffer ourselves from direct exposure to all the possibilities we could be pursuing. In truth, the degree of dynamic initiative we could be taking regardless of our life circumstances is limitless. *Are you willing to run out of excuses for moving toward your heart's desire?* is the question. Where can you skip the need for approval today and respond to what is being called for in your world by declaring a vision and intention for action?

Admitting how we're just playing it safe, using the excuse of not having permission, is a crucial step if we wish to start engaging our lives with purpose.

Beta Test Responses From Participants

There are some things that I have been wanting to do for a while now and I just keep waiting for "things to fall into place." Looking at the list, I realize that I need to just give my permission to go ahead—to not be afraid of making mistakes, because I can always learn from them and if I wait for things to happen—well, I could wait forever. —AG

This makes me face my biggest fears about some things I have wanted to do but was afraid to start and, yes, it would include my husband's input and support. Thank you for helping me put it down on paper and naming it—that makes me look at it and puts it out there for me to see. —BW

The list I made today was more of a bucket type wish list—not anything that needs to get done today or this week. The only one stopping me from doing any of these items is myself. So I gave myself

*permission to dream about making different choices
than I am currently making and think about how
my life would be different. I find that I get so busy
that I don't slow down to think about getting out of
the rut and what that would feel like. —SG*

*Well, that was hard and scary. And totally exhil-
arating! I feel most alive when I'm staring at my
true heart's-desire in the face. It's amazing how
something so tactical and tangible as a list can lead
me straight to my core. —RD*

Developing Confidence of Creativity
Game 4 – Games for Confidence
Move toward Chaos

This practice is to move toward a circumstance or situation
that feels chaotic to you. We often call any potent
expression of energy that is new, unfamiliar, or difficult to
control "chaotic." It could be a room full of kids, a concert
crowd, a space that hasn't been organized, a parade, a
project with many elements, a trading floor, a convention,
our own desk, or a city street we have to navigate to get
somewhere. Situations that we feel we may lose control
in are perfect environments for getting face to face with
our stress precedents. The ability or willingness to tolerate

chaotic energy or circumstances opens us up to a whole range of opportunities we are otherwise bound to miss. In addition, the circumstances and domains we label as "chaotic" often represent where the most energy is. We can draw juice for creative and dynamic progression in our lives from these circumstances.

As you move toward a chaotic circumstance that you usually avoid, make up a new story that is useful to you. "I'm going to learn something here" is an example of a useful belief. "Whatever happens here, I can handle it" is another.

Beta Test Responses from Participants

I had to make a two-hour trip from my home to catch a flight today. I missed it due to border traffic, a highway accident, and an insane amount of rush hour traffic. All the way along, my impulse was to simply call off the meeting I was heading to, turn around, go home and be in my calm and predictable house with my family. I kept driving, however, and reaching the airport was able to find an alternate red-eye flight to get where I needed to go. It feels like some kind of inner triumph to have moved through a circumstance like this I would ordinarily avoid. —RL

I decided to take this on and jump into chaos. Today's opportunity was to walk with a throng of students between classes. Normally, I would wait until the rush was over or choose a different, quieter path. This time I walked with the throng of students as they were hurrying to their class. It was certainly different for me and I enjoyed the energy I felt from the youth. It made me wonder what goals they are racing toward to be so committed to this activity. —KM

DEVELOPING CONFIDENCE OF EFFORT
Game 5 – Games for Confidence
Make No Excuses

The vast majority of the excuses we give for not following through on something—for failing to complete, step up to, handle, or take responsibility for something—are actually just a cover-up for giving in to a stress reaction. Try making *absolutely no excuses* today, even if you have the most legitimate one in the world. In the space where your defense would have stood, commit to taking just one small step forward. We don't know what amazing results may be set in motion by even one small, right effort.

Our excuse might be that we have too much to do and don't know where to start. Again, identifying and committing to one small step is a practice of *intelligent misbehavior*. Paradoxically, having too many steps in front of us dilutes the focus of our commitments and shields us from being responsive to them. As *Good to Great* author Jim Collins says, "When you have more than three priorities, you don't have any."[1] What we do have is a rich breeding ground for excuses.

Beta Test Responses from Participants

This "no excuses" practice is a very good reminder for me and I really appreciated Jim Collins' quote regarding the necessity to define priorities. I find that I frequently fail to define my top priorities, and even when I attempt to, I can be easily distracted by the many tantalizing opportunities that abundantly present themselves. I also have been known to verbalize my excuses, which frankly is not a very becoming method of communication. Just this morning, I found myself starting to state an excuse and rather than elucidating upon the details of it, if not initially embracing the suggested silence, I trailed off and my audience obviously didn't mind!—KT

Yikes! I'm an excuse-maker. I tend to make excuses not only for myself, but for my people, as well.

Self-defense, protect the EGO at all costs! I had a long day. I had to take blame, and responsibility and such. However, as it turns out, people rather respected this. I was pleasantly surprised, and on my way to a new "habit." Thank you for this one!—JD

I learned that justifications don't have to be ver-balized. When a task came up that required real analysis (not just associative thought) I found myself "vegging" or "stalling" by getting distracted by reading some news articles. This is actually a normal part of my job: to read the tech and security news to keep abreast of developments. However, as I am learning, anything "good" can be used as an excuse for something "bad." So twice yesterday I caught myself doing that and brought my atten-tion back to the task at hand and held it there until I got past the sticking point. Once my mind engaged, there was momentum and fun energy to keep going—it's just getting through those initial minutes requiring focus and will power.—KC

Aarrggh! I really dislike reading some of these [comments] and thinking, "hmmm, that sounds familiar." It makes me uncomfortable. I've been putting many to-do items ahead of one that really needed to get done this week. I absolutely knew why I was doing that and avoiding it only made me think about it more. More often than not it's never as hard, bad, time consuming as I've built it up to be and that was true in this case. I cleared it off my desk this morning.—TW

CONFIDENCE LEADS TO RELATIONSHIP

My son was a passionate hockey player when we lived in Canada. When we moved to the southwestern United States, he joined a recreational hockey league in Arizona, which, being short on ice, relied upon outdoor sports courts and inline roller skates instead of Zambonis and traditional ice skates for its play. Practices and pickup games took place on the grounds of a new outdoor facility in the small town where we lived at the time, and parents would routinely bring their youngsters to the complex, drop them off for a few hours of recreation, then return later to pick them up. I always felt a little hesitant to do this, since hockey isn't the most benign of sports. As a result, I would often bring work with me and sit in my car in the parking lot near the open rink where I could view the kids' activities without hovering too conspicuously.

I'm not the first parent to have to manage the stress of getting his kid to sports practices and get work done on the side, but I was finding it particularly challenging to stay focused on the book I was writing at the time and also keep up with getting my son to his activities.

There was one other parental figure who regularly remained for these sessions. He was the grandfather of a good friend of my son. His name was Doyle. Doyle was a physical tower of Southern charm, warm and sweet to the kids. He had spent most of his life in Oklahoma and spoke with an accent that was thicker than cough syrup. You might think that as a comedian, entertainer, and speaker I'd be an outgoing person by nature, but it's pretty much the opposite. I'm a good measure of introvert, often preferring quiet solitude, internal reflection, and individual creative work and focus.

On this day, as usual, I turned off the social switch and buried myself in my own writing work. The book I was working on was *7 Rules You Were Born to Break*, which is all about breaking one's own unconscious rules.[2] As was regularly the case, the grandfather and I were sitting in our separate vehicles while the boys scrimmaged. I was getting lots of work done, and Doyle, the grandpa, was unoccupied.

I noticed the kind elder sitting patiently, watching his grandson with affection and waiting for the game to conclude. I was often moved by his devotion to his grandson but, quite frankly, did not go out of my way to get into lengthy conversations with him, despite his being the accepting gentleman that he was. The fact is, I find social interactions themselves stressful. It really doesn't matter who they're with. On this day, however, I found my attention being drawn toward Doyle—and I tried to ignore it. Yet, I was writing about one of the "rules" we follow: the human tendency to pretend we don't matter, and the fact that we need to break this rule if we wish to reach our full potential.

Pretending we don't matter is a behavior that is built on the belief that we can't make a difference—perhaps a holdover from childhoods where we were raised to be "seen, but not heard." It's not true, of course. Every last one of us matters. Yet, believing that we don't, it's tempting to hide out and hold back, because hiding out allows us to temporarily avoid the stress of showing up in human relationships.

The irony of my position—writing to encourage others to do the very thing I was ignoring—did not escape me. I looked over at Doyle again. The demonstration of his heartfelt attention on the kids was a shining example of mattering to his grandson. As I looked at him sitting in his pickup truck, staring at the rink, a deeper instinct was calling out to me to engage with him, yet the stress involved with connecting left me wanting to stay holed up and just get things done. I tried to go back to my work, but I couldn't shake the thought that I should stop writing about this topic and actually engage it. I wrestled for a while with my lack of confidence in engaging others and the obvious need for it.

I got out of my vehicle the way a four-year-old finally responds to his mother when she won't stop nagging him to get out of the house and go play. "Okaaay!" my inner child whined, as I put away my laptop, got out of the car, and walked around the back of Doyle's pickup to approach him from the driver's side and say hello. Strolling up alongside his window, I stood just next to the left rearview mirror and waited for him to notice I was there. But he didn't. He just continued to stare straight ahead at the rink. Finally, I tapped lightly on the glass. He then slowly turned to look at me, seeming a little confused. I had to prompt him to roll down the window, which he did, cracking it open enough that we could converse.

We started to talk as I asked him the usual "how are you" kind of questions, and Doyle responded with a run of phrases that were typically hard for me to decipher due to the flavor of his Southern delivery. I managed to keep the conversation going as I caught a few of his words, but as our dialogue continued I realized that his accent was not the only barrier. The actual content of his speech involved some odd concepts and indicated that he was feeling stressed and disoriented. Indeed, after a few minutes he managed to articulate that he was feeling funny.

Getting a little concerned, I asked him for more details and to roll down the window the rest of the way so I could properly hear him. As he attempted to do as I asked, it became apparent that his left arm wasn't functioning. He had to bring his right arm across his chest to complete the task. It then dawned on me what was happening. I called 911 immediately and explained that the older gentleman I was with might be having a stroke.

As luck would have it, an ambulance had stationed itself on call at a high school soccer game on the other side of the same park. Arriving less than two minutes later, the paramedics confirmed that a stroke had occurred and worked very quickly to get Doyle out of the vehicle and into the ambulance. He was in the emergency room within ten minutes of his stroke.

Doyle outlived that fateful day by many years, enjoying his loving family as a functional person with minimal damage to his brain and nervous system. Even a minute more of a delay between his stroke and his reaching the hospital would have left him far worse off, and potentially he would not have lived through the event. Every time I see Doyle's daughter, the mother of my son's friend, she credits me with saving her father's life. I didn't have a commitment to save a life, however. I only had a small commitment to play confidence-building games, to stretch into unfamiliar territory and challenge my fears a little bit. More often than we might think, that small commitment can have enormous benefit to ourselves and to others.

GAMES FOR CONFIDENCE PLATFORM

The standard ways of coping with stress are to try to deal with it privately and alone, attempting to reduce or eliminate the triggers of our anxiety. Applied intentionally, this can be healthy and useful. Applied as a blanket measure, however, we eliminate many opportunities to stretch beyond our current comfort zone and enrich our life engagement. Avoidance of stress, as a rule, shrinks our lives and leaves the stress-reaction habit fully intact, like landmines from an old war that we could step on at any time.

None of us can make stress go away. Even if we never left our own home, we'd still have to deal with the intrusion of mind—of our personal past upon our present experience. Besides, an isolated life would be sad, because you can't contribute to other human beings without relating to them—and living our highest point of contribution is what is going to heal us. Wanting to make a positive contribution gives us the necessity to transform the presence of stress in our lives into rocket fuel.

Since the 1970s, many people have learned, through mindfulness training and other avenues of healing, to free themselves from toxic stress. Many have adopted healthier lifestyles. We couldn't claim, however, that these healthier habits pervade the atmosphere of mainstream culture. There is still a cultural inertia where many of us create toxic stress through our lifestyles and then relieve the symptoms of the stress with behavior that only puts a Band-Aid on the wound. This necessitates dealing with these same stresses over and over again.

Fortunately, we have an alternative. Our own dedication to our best lives through consistent, reliable, small-scale efforts that we can make day in and day out and sustain over time is that alternative. This dedication will bring real results and get us where we want to go without triggering old defense systems and derailing the progress we're making.

Growing in confidence requires making sure there isn't *too much* stress, or *too little* stress, present at any given time. Just like the old analogy about a musical instrument requiring the right amount of tension on the strings to make music: not too tight and not too loose. Our cultural reaction to stress is to loosen the strings as much as possible, but that doesn't inspire the music we're capable of creating as a human being. What's missing in the *too much/too little* equation is an understanding of stress *production*—how to keep the right amount and type of stress present and use it as fuel for creativity, expression, passion, great relationships, profit, entrepreneurship, leadership, art, innovation, fertile corporate culture, health, beauty, and all the human endeavors that require large amounts of energy to thrive. We can get that energy from the creative tension of productive stress, if we learn how to harvest it.

I've described my belief that *intelligent misbehavior* —awareness of old limits accompanied by courageous action—practiced in the midst of our daily lives is the real answer to change. This awareness is also the key to overcoming anxiety and staying in forward motion with useful action.

The five *Games for Confidence* I've shared here are a few examples of hundreds more that I share on my training site at: *www.gamesforconfidence.com.* I invite you to visit me there and find out how you can use the games to fully thrive in a community atmosphere with like-minded individuals inspiring each other to respond confidently to the challenges of life.

Between stimulus and response there's a space. In that space is our power to choose our response. In our response lies our growth and our freedom.
—Victor Frankl

PART FIVE

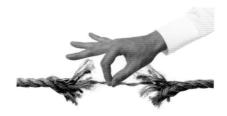

MY PERSONAL STRUGGLE WITH CONFIDENCE

TO THE BRINK OF BANKRUPTCY

Many of you will remember the business collapse of 2009, the year the bottom fell out of the stock market, bankruptcies soared by 32 percent and everything involving business seemed to come to a screeching halt.

While the entire economy was dealt a big blow, the meeting industry was hit even harder after a few high-profile corporations were publicly criticized for spending shareholder money on "unnecessary" special events at that time. Understandably, many other companies decided not to risk such critical perceptions of their own organizations until things had calmed down. The result was the mass cancellation of planned business gatherings and conferences.

The experience for me and for many industry peers and colleagues—event planners, speakers bureaus, entertainment agencies, hotels, and all forms of meeting suppliers—was unprecedented and devastating, even for those of us who had been in the industry for decades and had seen many economic cycles come and go before. But never like this. I didn't know it at the time, but my phone wouldn't ring for the next six months. All I knew was that our bank account was shrinking, month by month—a one-way outflow of expenses with no replenishment.

With two children from a previous marriage and my wife in her first trimester of pregnancy with our first child together, I watched her belly grow, my family of four about to become a family of five. And not a stitch of work was in sight. Like millions of others at that time I was worried; losing more and more confidence in myself and in the situation day by day.

As a self-employed entertainer, I had learned the basics of web design in order to market my services online. I lived in a small town at the time and started pounding the local pavement, walking into shops and stores to see if I might convince a few small business owners to invest in an online presence by hiring me to create a website for their company. I was successful enough to keep us afloat and started getting better at web design. I enjoyed helping business owners tell their story by defining the essence of their unique value and communicating that offering in words and pictures. As had many others, I'd taken a very large pay cut to find work, but I was relieved to have measurably slowed the draining of our reserves. In fact, I started to think about what it would take to make a profit by dedicating myself to this new profession.

I shared these thoughts with my wife. I told her about the success I was having and some of the ways I imagined this design business could grow. I shared my fears regarding our finances and the relief I was feeling in discovering this new potential. As she listened to me make my case, I imagined she was sharing my feeling of relief. But when she spoke, what she said surprised me. Not just her words, but the force behind them—a force that would change my work and the course of our lives together in a dramatic way.

She began by saying that she understood my thinking and that it made sense logically in the face of our circumstances. "And," she added, "I forbid you to become a web designer!" Then she stopped and waited for my brain to catch up. This was not what I expected from the mouth of a pregnant woman. "That's not what you are here for," she continued. "You were born to be in front of audiences, to make them laugh, to entertain them, to lift people up and to inspire them. That's what you are here to do, and all you need to do is commit to that. That's our future!"

Her response blindsided me. I had been called out, confronted for playing small, and at the same time given a huge vote of confidence by my wife. She had looked straight past all my good reasons for switching professions, past the salesman in me dangling the promise of a secure future, and held who I really am—and who I am not—in a fierce and loving demand. "You are not a web designer," she concluded.

I was both exhilarated and scared by what she was standing for. On the surface, my fear was concern for our survival, a fear I could have justifiably defended. Underneath, however, was an unconscious reaction. The truth was, I was afraid of something that I had been ignoring—a larger calling and a sensed potential that I could offer something more to my audiences. That "something more" was a role as a professional speaker.

This would be a turning point out of the safety zone that I mentioned earlier. All my work to this point had been as a silent comedian, miming and mugging and circus tricks. Even the waiter character was silent, and it had all worked beautifully up to now. Yet, secretly, I had watched for years while motivational speakers and trainers educated and inspired the same groups I entertained, while thinking to myself, "I could do that if I wanted to." But truthfully, I was scared and unsure that I'd be able to pull it off. I wanted to be done with fear, and here it was again, my old friend in spades!

I was holding back on the opportunity to engage the passionately committed life that I wordlessly encouraged my audiences to embrace. I wanted to put words, inspiring stories, and understandable guidance into language and share what I loved about overcoming fear and living with confidence. Yet I had ignored that inspiration and had been suffering from exactly what I wanted to help others to transcend. There was no question that now was the time to stand for this possibility.

My wife knew it, had spoken it clearly, and now I could feel it, too. At the same time, the idea of moving toward this new potential felt extremely stressful—so much so that the current state of familiar stress looked more attractive than the prospect of the unknown. And even by logical standards, it made no sense. It was a crazy commitment in light of our circumstances and the state of the event industry. There were no guarantees. I would need to reinvent myself as a presenter of ideas and content relevant to businesses and corporations that were currently at *zero spend* for those services, competing with hordes of other speaking candidates looking for work. Needless to say, it was a huge challenge—and also undeniably the right path to commit to.

REBIRTH

Spring, 2009. My wife encouraged me to take advantage of the downtime to fully commit to developing the new material that could take my career to an entirely new level. With the enormous benefit of her support and with nothing but time on my hands, I took the opportunity to engage in an intense period of writing and reflection to find the language that would convey what I believed in. Yes, I was writing for others, but I had to inspire myself more than anyone to rise to this occasion. I was birthing myself into uncharted territory.

I sat at my desk and committed to write. For months on end, I wrote for eight, ten, twelve hours a day, recording the amazing stories and incidents of my performing and life experience. I searched for a theme I could authentically stand on. What did I really have to say? What did I know about? And what would I have the courage to demonstrate? After months of generating a list of over three hundred potential titles for this collection of writings, I stumbled upon the precise language needed to communicate my new profession. I was a *professional misbehaver*. A title for my new book effortlessly followed, and *7 Rules You Were Born to Break* came into existence. These 7 were rules that I personally needed to break if I was going to make it through this tunnel, and I followed my own advice while I recorded them, just to keep moving forward.

With no guarantees that this new approach would be accepted or marketable to the meeting industry, I just kept pouring out my thoughts and stories. The book took shape slowly, but I stuck with it and eventually finished. I began to communicate my new offering as a speaker, along with my entertainment, to customers and clients, old and new. Work began to materialize and a light appeared at the end of the tunnel. The following year would produce nearly double the income I had ever earned in a single year, despite a still sluggish economy. Business grew exponentially, and continues to grow, as a result of finally walking my talk.

Fear and doubt had almost convinced me to walk away from one of the most important opportunities of my life. My wife and I have always held each other accountable for not caving in to our self-doubts and fears. I have held her up and she has held me up. We live in an atmosphere where we challenge each other to keep our head above reactive patterns. Because of the work we do together, and her confident support in this instance, I was able to act from a position of response.

Confident Under Pressure is not, however, about my success. It's about what I almost walked away from, and about what you might be walking away from today in your life. This book is about the daily struggle that is required to walk *toward* instead of *away from* what is possible, and about the responsibility and opportunity we all face as human beings to keep our highest possibility alive. This coming alive, and staying alive, is a lifelong process and commitment. We need sources of inspiration and partners in practice to do it successfully.

If you have a wish to walk toward the greatest opportunities of your life that are often hidden in the ordinary stresses and challenges of your daily routine, you'll need two things:

1. An established practice of engaging challenges in small ways so you can build your capacity for confidence over time.

2. A network of support from like-minded individuals who can help you remember your aim to practice *intelligent misbehavior*.

If you'd like to get more support for living with confidence and turning the challenges of each ordinary day into a lifetime of extraordinary growth, visit my training site at www.gamesforconfidence.com. That's a way you can keep in touch and connect with others who are looking for mutual support to fully thrive in the human game.

You start dying slowly
if you do not travel,
if you do not read,
If you do not listen to the sounds of life,
If you do not appreciate yourself.
You start dying slowly
When you kill your self-esteem;
When you do not let others help you.
You start dying slowly
If you become a slave of your habits,
Walking everyday on the same paths…
If you do not change your routine,
If you do not wear different colours
Or you do not speak to those you don't know.
You start dying slowly
If you avoid to feel passion
And their turbulent emotions;
Those which make your eyes glisten
And your heart beat fast.
You start dying slowly
If you do not change your life when you are not
    satisfied with your job, or with your love,
If you do not risk what is safe for the uncertain,
If you do not go after a dream,
If you do not allow yourself,
At least once in your lifetime,
To run away from sensible advice…

                    —Martha Medeiros

acknowledgements

The books I've written, including this one, would never have come into being without the confidence that was instilled in me by my spiritual teacher, Lee Lozowick. He embodied confidence itself, demonstrating what it looks like to wear confidence in daily life—like a robe of faith rather than a suit of armor—conducting his own life with unshakable presence, to which I will forever aspire.

This book would also not have been possible without the generous support of my wife Clelia. Her companionship, love, clarity, sense of humor, support in letting me spend the long hours playing with words and willingness to call me back when I've lost my way have all been invaluable to me.

My thanks to my three children Nate, Ruby and Aditya who have tolerated the endless starts and stops of my million ideas and writing projects over the years, my extensive travels, and my sometimes less than confident and effective parenting. Still, I love you all beyond measure.

Thanks to my dear friends, editors and publishing team at Hohm Press: Regina Sara Ryan, Nancy Lewis, Dasya Zuccarello, Bala Zuccarello and Becky Fulker.

The quality of their care, guidance, attention and professionalism are unparalleled in the publishing industry. I am blessed as an author to have their support.

Thanks to all my early readers who provided their feedback and input on numerous versions and re-writes of this book: Bob Krieckhaus, Tarini Bauliya, Bob Ell, Michael Menager, Skye Burn, Geoff Carr and Richard Lewis. A special thanks to Tarini for challenging me to let my readers in "behind the scenes" of my own vulnerabilities in stress.

Thanks to the clients and meeting attendees who have given me the opportunity to speak to thousands of people about the ideas in this book, allowing me to test, refine and develop these ideas in a practical and useful way.

A final special thank you to Martha Meideros who generously granted permission for her poem, "A Morte Devagar," (A Slow Death), to appear at the end of my book. The poem was written in 2000 and has for a long time been erroneously attributed to Pablo Neruda. It is my wish that she enjoys the recognition that she deserves for this inspiring poem and that the text leading up to its appearance here emboldens every reader to "risk what is safe for the uncertain."

enpnotes

PART one:

1. Abiola Keller, Kristin Litzelman, Lauren E. Wisk, Torsheika Maddox, Erika Rose Cheng, Paul D. Creswell, and Whitney P. Witt, "Does the Perception that Stress Affects Health Matter? The Association with Health and Mortality," National Institute of Health, Sep 31, 2012, *https://www.ncbi.nlm.nih.gov/pmc/articles/PMC3374921/*

2. Mom.me Staff, "Funny Kids' Test Answers," *Mom.me*, Sep 20, 2016, *https://mom.me/kids/little-kid/6437-funny-kids-test-answers/item first-cells-were-probably/*

3. Daniel Kahneman, "The Riddle of Experience vs. Memory," *Ted Talk Video*, 19:57, Feb 2010, *https://www.ted.com/talks/daniel_kahneman_the_riddle_of_experience_vs_memory#t-1187370*

4. Professor Mohd Razali Salleh, MD, Oct 2008, "Life Event, Stress and Illness." *https://www.ncbi.nlm.nih.gov/pmc/articles/PMC3341916/*

5. Steve Nguyen, PhD, "Cost of Stress on the US Economy is 300 Billion, Says Who?" July, 2016. *https://workplacepsychology.net/2016/07/04/cost-of-stress-on-the-u-s-economy-is-300-billion-says-who/.* (The author of this article tracks down the original reference for what has become a much cited statistic regarding the cost of stress in the workplace. In the final analysis he shows why the number (300 billion) is to be taken with a grain (bucket?) of salt. The background calculations, however, of how the number was derived do make it clear there is a big cost to stress, though the exact number is perhaps unknowable.)

6. National Institute of Mental Health. "Social anxiety disorders". (2010) *http://www.nimh.nih.gov/health/publications/social-phobia*

7. Dave Scott, "Untitled," *American Way Magazine*, July 2016 Issue, 26.

8. Dr. Gabor Mate, "The Healing Force Within," *DrGaborMate.com*, Aug 15, 2013, *https://drgabormate.com/healing-force-within/*

9. Gay Hendricks, *The Big Leap*, NY: HarperOne™, 2009, 63.

10. Lee Rainie and Kathryn Zickuhr, "Americans' Views on Mobile Etiquette," Pew Research Center, Aug 26, 2015, *http://www.pewinternet.org/2015/08/26/americans-views-on-mobile-etiquette/*

PART TWO:

1. David Hoffeld, "Want to Know What Your Brain Does When It Hears a Question?" *FastCompany.com*, Feb 21, 2017, *https://www.fastcompany.com/3068341/want-to-know-what-your-brain-does-when-it-hears-a-question*

2. Peter Levine, *Waking the Tiger*, Berkeley, Calif.: North Atlantic Books, 1997, 34.

3. Op.cit., 6.

4. Amelia Aldao Ph.D, "Why Labeling Emotions Matters," *PsychologyToday.com*, Aug 4, 2014, *https://www.psychologytoday.com/blog/sweet-emotion/201408/why-labeling-emotions-matters*

5. Ortony and Turner, "Basic Emotions," *ChangingMinds.org*, *http://changingminds.org/explanations/emotions/basic%20emotions.htm*

6. Levine, 76.

7. Susan David, "How Achieving Emotional Agility Can Help You—at Work and at Life," *Knowledge@Wharton*, Oct 26, 2016, *http://knowledge.wharton.upenn.edu/article/how-achieving-emotional-agility-can-help-you-at-work-and-in-life/*

8. Dan Siegel, "Name It to Tame It," *YouTube*, Dec 8, 2014, *https://www.youtube.com/watch?v=ZcDLzppD4Jc*

9. Chris Helder, *Useful Belief*, Singapore: Wiley, 2016, 78.

10. Martin Sheen and Amy Goodman, "It Was the Happiest Day of My Life," *DemocracyNow.com*, May 2, 2016, *https://www.democracynow.org/2016/5/2/it_was_the_happiest_day_of*

11. Naomi Klein, *This Changes Everything*, New York: Simon & Schuster, 2014

PART THREE:

1. Wikipedia, "Yerkes-Dodson Law," Feb 8, 2018, *https://en.wikipedia.org/wiki/Yerkes%E2%80%93Dodson_law*

2. Dr. Geoffrey Carr, *Making Happiness*, Vancouver, BC: Geoffrey Carr, 2014. *http://drgeoffreycarr.com/making-happiness/*

3. Sian Beilock, *Choke*, New York: Simon & Shuster, 2010, 34.

4. Op. cit., 43.

5. Op. cit., 58.

6. Dr. Gabor Mate, "The Healing Force Within," *DrGaborMate.com*, Aug 15, 2013, *https://drgabormate.com/healing-force-within/*

7. Wikipedia, "Eustress," Jan 4, 2018, *https://en.wikipedia.org/wiki/Eustress*

8. Carol Dweck, "Carol Dweck Revisits the 'Growth Mindset'", *EdWeekorg*, Sep 22, 2015, *https://www.edweek.org/ew/articles/2015/09/23/carol-dweck-revisits-the-growth-mindset.html*

9. Justin Menkes, "How Stress Can Improve Your Performance," *HBR.org*, Ap 28, 2011, *https://hbr.org/2011/04/dont-let-stress-break-your-per*

10. Susan Fowler, *Why Motivating People Doesn't Work and What Does*, San Francisco: Berrett-Koehler Publishers, 2014, 42.

11. Stephen Guise, "My Life Changing Experience in a Deprivation Tank," *StephenGuise.com*, *http://stephenguise.com/my-life-changing-experience-in-a-sensory-deprivation-tank-my-review-after-six-floats-in-eight-days/*

12. Charles Duhigg, *The Power of Habit*, USA: Anchor Canada, 2012, 100.

13. Jim Corbett, "The Art of Smack," *UsaToday.com*, Jan 27, 2014, *https://www.usatoday.com/story/sports/nfl/super/2014/01/27/super-bowl-trash-talk-warren-sapp-keyshawn-johnson-terrell-suggs-shannon-sharpe--richard-sherman/4947983/*

14. Ryan Wilson, "#TBT: That Time When Shannon Sharpe Made Derrick Thomas Lose It," *CBSsports.com*, Sep 15, 2015, *https://www.cbssports.com/nfl/news/tbt-that-time-when-shannon -sharpe-made-derrick-thomas-lose-it/*

PART FOUR:

Kimberly Weisul, "Jim Collins: Good to Great in 10 Steps," *Inc.com*, May 7, 2012, *https://www.inc.com/kimberly-weisul/jim-collins- good-to-great-in-ten-steps.html*

Rick Lewis, *7 Rules You Were Born to Break: How Intelligent Misbehavior Can Help You and Your Organization Thrive,* Vancouver, BC: Break a Rule Publishing, 2010.

BIBLIOGRAPHY

Aldao, Amelia, Ph.D. "Why Labeling Emotions Matters." *PsychologyToday.com.* Aug 4, 2014.

Arbinger Institute. *Leadership and Self-Deception.* Oakland, Calif.: Berrett-Koehler Publishers, 2002.

Beilock, Sian. *Choke.* New York: Simon & Schuster, 2010.

Brown, Peter C., Mark A. McDaniel, and Henry L Roediger III. *Make it Stick.* Cambridge, Mass.: Harvard University/ Belknap Press, 2014.

Buckingham, Marcus and Curt Coffman. *First, Break All the Rules.* New York: Pocket Books, 1999.

Cardoso, John Paulo and Ken Tencer. *Cause a Disturbance.* New York: Morgan James Publishing, 2014.

Carr, Geoffrey, Ph.D. "Making Happiness." Vancouver, BC: Geoffrey Carr, 2014. http://drgeoffreycarr.com/ making-happiness/.

Christensen, Clayton M., Jeff Dyer, and Hal Gregersen. *The Innovator's DNA.* Grand Haven, Mich.: Brilliance Audio, 2014.

Cialdini, Robert, Noah Goldstein, and Steve J. Martin. *The Small Big.* New York: Grand Central Publishing, 2014.

Collins, Jim. *Good to Great.* New York: HarperBusiness, 2001.

Corbett, Jim. "The Art of Smack." *UsaToday.com.* Jan 27, 2014.

David, Susan. "How Achieving Emotional Agility Can Help You—at Work and at Life." *Knowledge@Wharton.* Oct 26, 2016.

Duhigg, Charles. *The Power of Habit.* Toronto: Anchor Canada, 2012.

Dunham, Bandhu Scott. *Creative Life.* Prescott, Ariz.: Hohm Press, 2005.

Dweck, Carol. "Carol Dweck Revisits the 'Growth Mindset." *EdWeekorg.* Sep 22, 2015.

Fowler, Susan. *Why Motivating People Doesn't Work and What Does.* Oakland, Calif.: Berrett-Koehler Publishers, 2014.

Goldsmith, Marshall. *What Got You Here Won't Get You There.* Hoboken, N.J.: Jossey Bass, 2011.

Guise, Stephen. *Mini Habits.* CreateSpace Independent Publishing Platform, 2013.

———. "My Life Changing Experience in a Deprivation Tank." *StephenGuise.com*

Hamilton, Diane Musho. *Everything Is Workable.* Boston: Shambhala Publications, 2013.

Harter, James K. and Rodd Wagner. *The 12 Elements of Great Managing.* Gallup Press, 2006.

Helder, Chris. *Useful Beliefs.* Singapore: Wiley, 2016.

Hendricks, Gay. *The Big Leap.* New York: HarperOne, 2009.

Hoffeld, David. *The Science of Selling.* Berkeley: TarcherPerigee, 2016.

———. "Want to Know What Your Brain Does When It Hears a Question?" *FastCompany.com.* Feb, 21, 2017.

Hollis, James. *What Matters Most.* New York: Avery, 2009.

Kahneman, Daniel. "The Riddle of Experience vs. Memory." *Ted Talk Video.* Feb 2010.

Keller, Abiola, Kristin Litzelman, Lauren E. Wisk, et al. "Does the Perception that Stress Affects Health Matter? The Association with Health and Mortality." *National Institute of Health*. Sept. 31, 2012. https://www.ncbi.nlm.nih.gov/pmc/articles/PMC3374921/.

Klein, Naomi. *This Changes Everything*. New York: Simon & Schuster, 2014.

Korb, Alex. *The Upward Spiral*. Oakland, Calif.: New Harbinger Publications, 2015.

Levine, Peter. *Waking the Tiger*. Berkeley, Calif.: North Atlantic Books, 1997.

Lewis, Rick. *7 Rules You Were Born to Break: How Intelligent Misbehavior Can Help You and Your Organization Thrive*. Vancouver, BC: Break a Rule Publishing, 2010.

Lozowick, Lee. *Just This 365*. Chino Valley, Ariz.: Hohm Press, 2017.

Mate, Dr. Gabor. "The Healing Force Within." *DrGaborMate.com*. Aug 15, 2013.

McRaney, David. *You Are Not So Smart*. New York: Avery, 2012.

Menkes, Justin. *Better Under Pressure*. Cambridge, Mass.: Harvard Business Review Press, 2011.

Menkes, Justin. "How Stress Can Improve Your Performance." *HBR.org*. Ap 28, 2011.

Moore, Susie. *What If It Does Work Out?* Dover/Ixia Press, 2017.

National Institute of Mental Health. "Social Anxiety Disorders." *National Institute of Mental Health*. 2010. *http://www.nimh.nih.gov/health/publicaitons/social-phobia*.

Nguyen, Steve, PhD, "Cost of Stress on the US Economy is 300 Billion, Says Who?" July, 2016, *WorkplacePsychology.net*

Ortony and Turner. "Basic Emotions." *ChangingMinds.org.* http://changingminds.org/explanations/emotions/basic%20 emotions.htm.

Rainie, Lee, and Kathryn Zickuhr. "Americans' Views on Mobile Etiquette." Pew Research Center. Aug 26, 2015. *http://www.pewinternet.org./2015/08/26/americans-view-on-mobile*-etiquette/.

Pink, David H. *A Whole New Mind.* New York: Riverhead Books, 2006.

Pressfield, Steven. *The War of Art.* Black Irish Books, 2012.

Razali Salleh, Mohd, MD, Oct 2008, "Life Event, Stress and Illness." https://www.ncbi.nlm.nih.gov/

Red Hawk. *Self Observation.* Prescott, Ariz.: Hohm Press, 2009.

Rubin, Gretchen. *Better Than Before.* New York: Broadway Books, 2015.

Scott, Dave. "Untitled." *American Way Magazine.* July 2016, Issue 26.

Sheen, Martin, and Amy Goodman. "It Was the Happiest Day of My Life." *DemocracyNow.com.* May 2, 2016.

Siegel, Dan. "Name It to Tame It." *YouTube.* Dec 8, 2014.

Sivers, Derek. *Anything You Want.* New York: Portfolio, 2015.

Staff, Mom.me. "Funny Kids' Test Answers." *Mom.me.* Sep 20, 2016.

Sunstein, Cass R.and Richard H. Thaler. *Nudge.* New York: Penguin Books, 2009.

Weisul, Kimberly. "Jim Collins: Good to Great in 10 Steps." *Inc. com*. May 7, 2012.

Wikipedia. "Yerkes-Dodson Law." *wikipedia.org*. Feb 8, 2018.

Wikipedia. "Eustress." *wikipedia.org.* Jan 4, 2018.

Wilson, Ryan. "#TBT: That Time When Shannon Sharpe Made Derrick Thomas Lose It." *CBSsports.com.* Sep 15, 2015.

INDEX

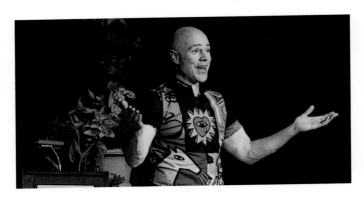

To check Rick's availability for speaking presentations, please visit:

www.ricklewis.co/presentations

~

All owners of this soft cover book are entitled to discounted pricing of the audio version of *Confident Under Pressure*, read by the author, Rick Lewis.

To order the audiobook version, please visit:

www.ricklewis.co/confidentunderpressure

~

For discount large-order purchases for groups and events, please visit:

www.ricklewis.co/confidentunderpressure/events

about the author

RICK LEWIS translates a lifetime of training in theater and comedy, spiritual practice, and professional development into the business realm, now using his knowledge to drive results for association and corporate professionals. He attended the Webster College Theater Conservatory before joining the national touring company of the Broadway musical *Barnum*, and has worked as a street performer, a comedian and speaker for corporate events, and a trainer in personal development for a nationally based seminar company. A longtime student of Lee Lozowick, Rick is the author of books on meditation, spiritual practice, and business development, including *7 Rules You Were Born to Break*, in which he shares his insights on "Intelligent Misbehavior" today with hundreds of Fortune 500 and other companies. Rick currently resides in Arizona with his wife and youngest child and continues in his dedication to spiritual and professional development in association with a small community of practitioners.

about hohm press

HOHM PRESS and affiliate Kalindi Press are committed to publishing books that provide readers with alternatives to the materialistic values of the current culture, and promote self-awareness, the recognition of interdependence, and compassion. Our subject areas (Hohm Press) include parenting, transpersonal psychology, religious studies, women's studies, the arts and poetry. And health, nutrition, family and children's books (Kalindi Press).

Contact Information: Hohm Press, PO Box 4410, Chino Valley, Arizona, 86323; USA; 800-381-2700, or 928-636-3331; email: *publisher@hohmpress.com*

Visit our websites at
www.hohmpress.com, www.kalindipress.com